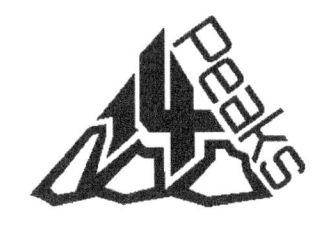

MEDICINE BALL WORKOUTS 8-WEEK FITNESS PLAN

Step-by-Step Instructions

for Medicine Ball Exercises

Copyright © 2017 14 PEAKS

MEDICINE BALL WORKOUTS

8-WEEK FITNESS PLAN

All rights reserved.

Published by 14 Peaks

Edited and formatted by 14 Peaks

Cover Design by Dunkin's Designs

ISBN-13: 978-1545462119

ISBN-10: 1545462119

This book is licensed for your personal enjoyment only. This book may not be re-sold or given away to other people. If you would like to share this book with another person, please purchase an additional copy for each person. If you're reading this book and did not purchase it, or it was not purchased for your use only, then please return it and purchase your own copy. Thank you for respecting the hard work of the authors.

Table of Contents

Introduction 1

Chapter 1: What Is a Medicine Ball? 3

Chapter 2: All about Medicine Balls 7

Chapter 3: How to Pick a Great Medicine Ball 11

Chapter 4: Getting Started with Your Workout 15

Chapter 5: Simple Medicine Ball Exercises 17

    Single Leg Slams 18

    Sit-Ups 20

    Lunge 22

    Pushups 24

    Overhead Squat 26

    Chest Pass 28

    Overhead Pass 30

    Overhead Lateral Bends 32

    Shoulder Press 34

    Supermans 36

Chapter 6: Intermediate Medicine Ball Exercises 39

    Lunge with Twist 40

    V-Ups 42

    Side Toss 44

Russian Twist 46

Woodchopper 48

Halo Slam 50

Staggered Pushup 52

Overhead Walking Lunge 54

Single Arm Chest Pass 56

Thruster 58

Chapter 7: Complex Medicine Ball Exercises 61

Wall Ball 62

Burpee Slams 64

In and Out Pushups 68

Alternating Pushups 70

Chest Pass to Pushups 72

Burpee Wall Ball 74

Lunge Slam 76

Sprinter Start Chest Pass 78

Squat Rockers 80

Dead Bugs 82

Chapter 8: 8-Week Workout Program 85

Conclusion 123

Introduction

This book is designed to give you a background of the medicine ball and focusses on step-by-step instructions for over 30 medicine ball exercises. By enlisting Sammy Parney, USA rugby player and graduate of the American Academy of Sports, you get detailed easy-to-understand instructions. Sammy also demonstrates each exercise, allowing you to see the proper form.

Not sure which muscle you're targeting? Each exercise is broken up with information on the primary and secondary muscles used for that exercise. There are tips to help you get the most out of each exercise.

Finally, there is an 8-week fitness plan for using your medicine ball. All you will need is a medicine ball and your body. The fitness plan is for total body fitness and works on strength and utilizes plyometrics to increase your power.

As a USA national team rugby player, Sammy understands the need for power, and she will teach you some of those same techniques. While there are many ways to do plyometrics and to work on power, the medicine ball is a great way to target your core and upper body, as well as your lower body for explosive speed.

Chapter 1
What Is a Medicine Ball?

A medicine ball is a weighted ball that is used for both fitness and therapy. Typically, it is about a shoulder's width wide, but the trend is towards larger ones ranging all the way up to 36 inches. The balls weigh between 2 to 300 pounds. Yes, you read that correctly! Some medicine balls weigh as much as 300 pounds, but the average workout ball is around 15 pounds. This of course depends on your strength and the purpose of the exercise.

Medicine balls come in all shapes and sizes and are made with various materials. You may also hear it referred to as an exercise, med or fitness ball.

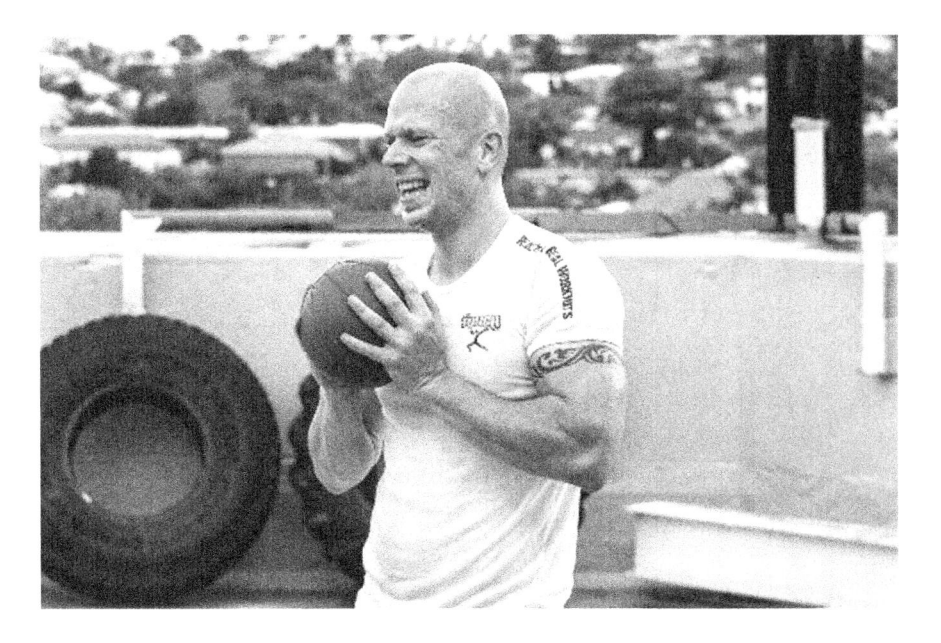

Why a Medicine Ball?

The medicine ball is widely used in the medical field, especially for sports medicine and physical therapy. It is also popular in strength training; CrossFit has really popularized the medicine ball.

In addition, the ball is excellent for kids and novices to use to get used to free-weight exercises. The medicine ball is very flexible and tends to mimic real-life movements, which makes it very popular.

Why Use a Medicine Ball?

Popular uses for the ball include:

- Physical therapy
- Strength training
- Fitness
- CrossFit
- Conditioning
- Speed training for muscles via plyometrics

A Little History

Somewhere around 400 BC, the ancient Greek physician Hippocrates is said to have employed the use of medicine balls with his patients to improve and to maintain good physical health. He believed using the medicine ball could cure a multitude of illness. Of course, we know it was the work not the actual ball. In those days, the balls were made of animal skins and were filled with sand. By the 19th century, the exercise balls were more like basketball shells filled with rags.

Medicine balls made a splash with sailors as far back as 1,000 BC. Persian soldiers used to fill bladders with sand for resistance training. Doctors told sailors to use them to combat seasickness and boredom when on ships.

There are various ideas about the origin of the word *medicine ball*. *Medicine* was originally synonymous with *health*. It was close in looks to the Native American term *medicine bag*, and thus the term *medicine ball* became popular.

President Hoover popularized the medicine ball with his game of "Hoover Ball." He wanted to lose some weight and started a new game. It was similar to volleyball, in that they used a volleyball net but with a medicine ball!

In 2001, the WallShot was popularized by CrossFit. It is a much hated move, only because it is so draining. The results speak for themselves, with gains in strength and power.

The Health Benefits of the Medicine Ball

The medicine ball gets its name honestly as it is a diverse therapeutic tool, not only for medicinal purposes but for getting in shape as well. The real beauty of exercising with the ball is how effective it is at involving a group of joints of muscles. It engages full body movements and resembles activities we do in our daily lives, which makes it a popular fitness tool for many populations.

Strength, power, agility and balance are a few of the areas the medicine ball can enhance.

The medicine ball is very popular for rehabilitating injuries but is also great for preventative measures. Regular use of the exercise ball will help keep your body fit and strong.

Some More Benefits of the Medicine Ball

- Minimal cost
- Minimal space required to use or store it
- Burns fat
- Builds muscle
- Improves coordination
- Promotes balance
- Increases power when done as plyometrics
- Is portable

Chapter 2
All about Medicine Balls

While the first known medicine balls were made of animal skins and were filled with sand, such is not the case anymore. The construction and materials that make up a medicine ball are as evolving as the ball itself. Let's take a look at the dynamics of the modern med ball.

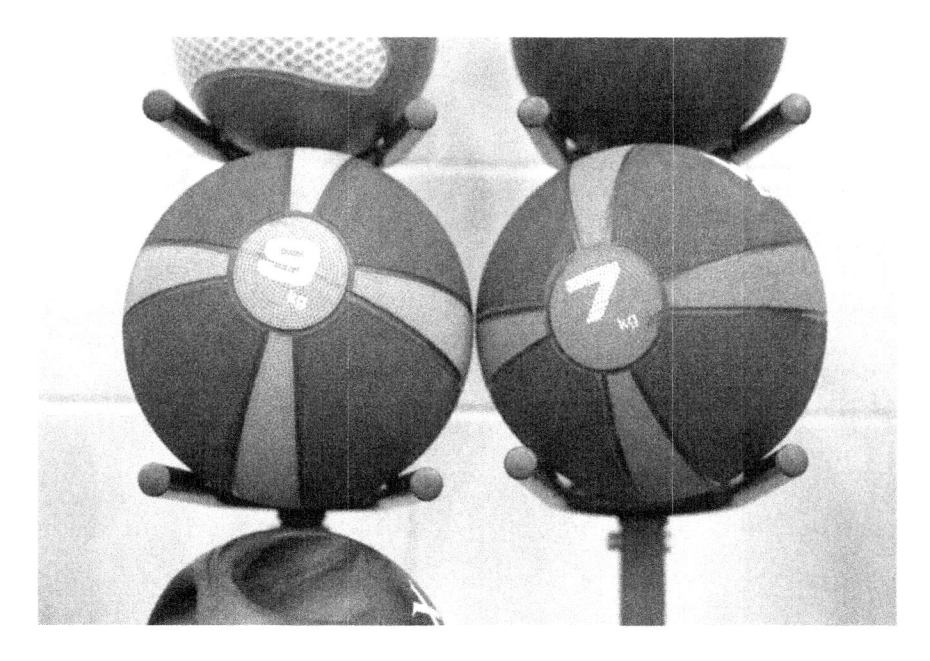

Types of Medicine Balls

The different types of medicine balls are designed with their application in mind. That is why there is such diversity of shapes, sizes and abilities when it comes to the exercise balls.

Some are quite small and serve well for hand-held exercises while others are larger and heavier for strength training. There are those that have handles or ropes. Some are designed with tough exteriors and grip easily while others are smooth for ease in catching.

Here is a look at some of the many types of medicine balls that are available:

Leather Medicine Balls

Leather is popular in the boxing arena and you may have even seen leather balls in old boxing movies or an old boxing match. Still, they are made today and the demand is plentiful so there is no indication they will be going away anytime soon. Century is very popular with this group and they have both leather and synthetic balls.

Grip Medicine Balls

For some exercises, you may want grips on the surface of the exercise ball. Most of the balls that do have such a grip are made of solid polyurethane. You will not need a ball with grips for the exercises in this book.

These balls usually have a small amount of bounce and are the most popular type of ball on the market, used by rehabs as well as gyms. The balls generally float as well, so they are widely used for water exercises and for conditioning for polo and aquatics.

Soft Gel Medicine Balls

Made of soft vinyl, the soft gel balls are filled with gel, just as the name implies. They are perfect for tossing and don't bounce if dropped. Neither do they float. Gel balls come in a good number of shapes and sizes and are a staple in rehabilitation facilities. They are also low cost.

Air-Filled Medicine Balls

Commonly used in plyometrics and resistance exercises, air-filled balls are great for those who want a lightweight ball that will bounce some. The more air they contain, the more they will bounce. They are easy to carry around and float too so they are great for a number of purposes, making a type of ball many gyms utilize.

Handled Medicine Balls

Medicine balls are often used for dynamic workouts, and a ball with a handle certainly comes in handy.

The handle is usually on one side, so it leaves one hand free and is not easily dropped during the active workout session. It is also excellent for exercises that call for using more than one ball, similar to those that use a kettlebell or dumbbell.

There are several advantages to using handled medicine balls during a workout, one being their ability to be used for explosive exercises. They are easier to handle in some cases than a dumbbell and especially a kettlebell.

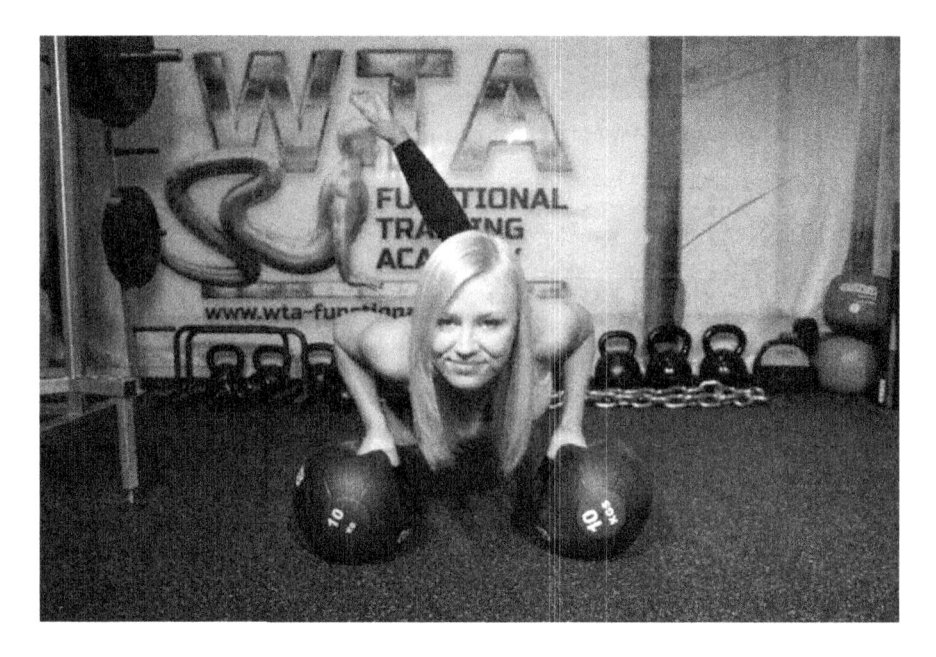

Some medicine ball handles are extended and the handles can be removed. The extendable ones generally go out about 12 inches in each direction. Some are designed for practicing a golf swing. While there is debate in the scientific community about using weighted equipment for specific sports, some still do it. Doug McGuff of *Body by Science* doesn't believe you should use weighted equipment for specific sports activities.

Medicine Balls with a Rope

You've probably seen the medicine balls that have a rope attached to them. Commonly the ropes can be detached but some are on permanently. These balls are great for swinging exercises and core rotation movements. They are great for core workouts.

There are even more types of medicine balls, but this group encompasses quite a large range.

Chapter 3
How to Pick a Great Medicine Ball

There are several factors that go into choosing a medicine ball. Below is a look at some things to consider when choosing a ball:

Purpose: Perhaps the most important thing to take into consideration is the purpose you will be using the ball for.

Size: Size does matter when it comes to medicine balls. The size of a ball makes a difference on the results you will get from it and what you can do with it, so be sure to find out the appropriate size for your needs. It is great to have a couple of sizes for various exercises.

Weight: Because the use of the medicine ball generally entails using multiple muscle groups that mimic how the body moves functionally, the rule of thumb is to start with a fairly lightweight ball. You may or may not work up to a heavier one, depending upon your purpose in your workout. Lighter weights are often used for toning, while heavier weights are used for strength training and power.

Construction: Construction can imply a number of aspects. Of course you want to get a medicine ball that is made of good quality. Some balls are made of slick material while others are designed to grip. You'll find nylon, leather, rubberized and a wide assortment of other materials. Believe it or not, some balls have beans in them.

The choice here can be the ball you prefer, as weight will be more important. Also be sure to consider the exercises you will be doing. For the exercises in this book you will need a medicine ball without handles or a rope and it can be smooth or have small grips on it.

Shape: The shape of the ball also goes along with what you will be doing with it. If you are using it in motion, you may need or want it to have a handle. There are elongated balls for certain exercises and others that have less air or are made of gel. Be sure you know the specifics before you go shopping.

What Is a Good Brand of Medicine Ball?

Amazon is a great place to go because you can see all the reviews. Here are our top five picks as far as brands go:

1. **The Valeo Medicine Ball** is a good pick, although it runs a little higher than most. It is of good quality and superb construction. It also retains its shape quite well.

2. In the squishy section, **ZoN oft Medicine Ball** is the best. It is small enough to work into many exercises and has a great, well-constructed design.

3. **Rep Fitness** is big in the CrossFit community, and they are hard on the medicine balls. It is a good quality ball that will last through those grueling workouts. This is a good ball for the workouts in this book.

4. **The Millard Double-Grip** is great for integration into many workouts such as core training ones. The grips are helpful when doing squats and lunges.

5. **Amazon** thrives on reviews and it has a money back guarantee. They have their own brand called **AmazonBasics,** which is good quality.

6. **Century** also makes a good medicine ball that our staff has used for years for CrossFit. It is popular among martial artists.

7. There are a myriad of medicine balls that would work, so don't feel tied down to these. These are just a few that we like.

Chapter 4
Getting Started with Your Workout

The exercises in this book are divided into simple and complex. Many of the exercises are plyometric exercises that will help with speed and strength, which equals power.

The explosive movements work on your power.

You will not need any other equipment besides the ball and your body. Talk about the perfect set up for minimalists! This also makes it a great workout if you travel a lot.

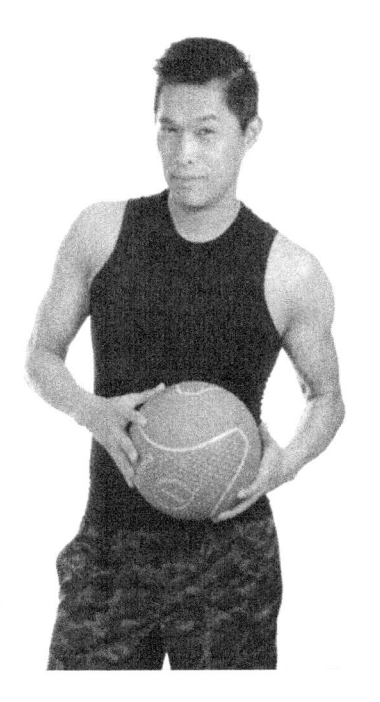

Points to Ponder:

- Plyometric exercises are intense, so work up to full speed.

- Our program will have 3-4 workouts per week, giving your body rest on the off days. Rest is when your body makes its muscular gains. You're actually growing your muscles when you're resting.

- We incorporate a rest week. You'll still workout but it will be light exercises to give your body a chance to rejuvenate.

- When you add body movements, such as jumping, you can exert up to seven times the force of your own bodyweight. Good shoes are important. CrossFit makes a shoe that's good for this type of workout; many cross trainers are great for this too.

Tips:

Here are some tips that will help assure you get the maximum benefits from your ball:

- Warm up before exercising with the med ball. We have warm-ups incorporated into the workouts.
- Start gradual and listen to your body.
- Technique is important to avoid injury.
- Get the technique right before you work on your speed.

Space

For some of the exercises, you need a wall. Our staff has used the brick walls of their home. It doesn't have to be fancy.

Workout Partner

Some medicine ball workouts require that you do them with a partner. The ones in the book do not. You can, however, grab a friend and workout together.

Chapter 5
Simple Medicine Ball Exercises

These are labeled as simple medicine ball exercises. That does not mean they are easy to do. They work the body hard. They are called simple in that they are single exercise and not as complex as some of the other exercises. Professionals as well as novices use these, so don't be fooled by the word simple.

SINGLE LEG SLAMS

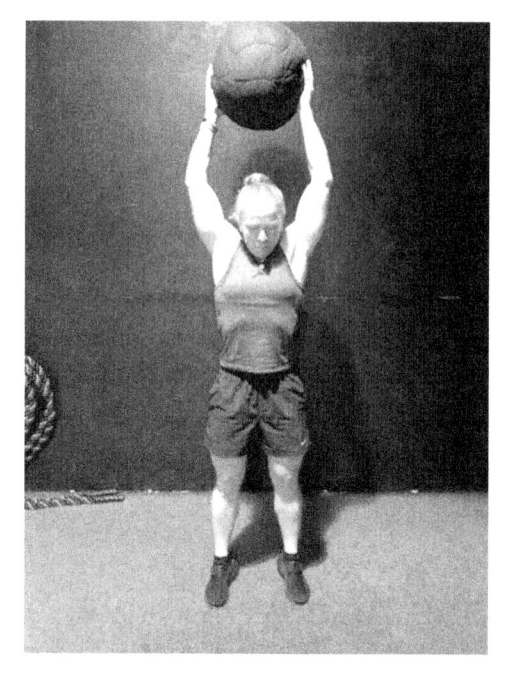

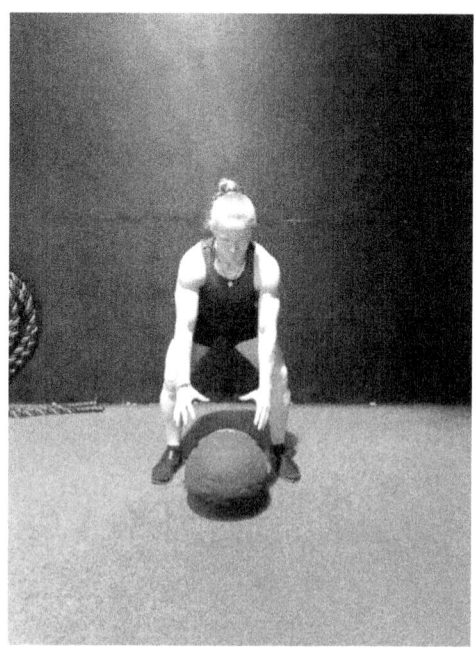

Slams: The medicine ball slam is the quintessential med ball exercise, and it is the foundation for other staple med ball exercises.

Primary muscles: Chest, abs

Secondary muscles: Shoulders, legs

Steps:

1. Stand with feet shoulder-width apart, holding the medicine ball overhead.

2. Forcefully throw the medicine ball to the ground, in front of your feet, contracting the abs and bringing the arms through, ending with the knees slightly bent.

3. If possible, catch the ball on the bounce. Otherwise, pick the medicine ball up from the ground and lift it back to the starting position, extending the arms overhead.

4. Repeat.

Keys: Start fully extended each time. Use as much force as possible in the slam, and be sure to contract the abs to keep the back from rounding.

Medicine Ball Workout

SIT-UPS

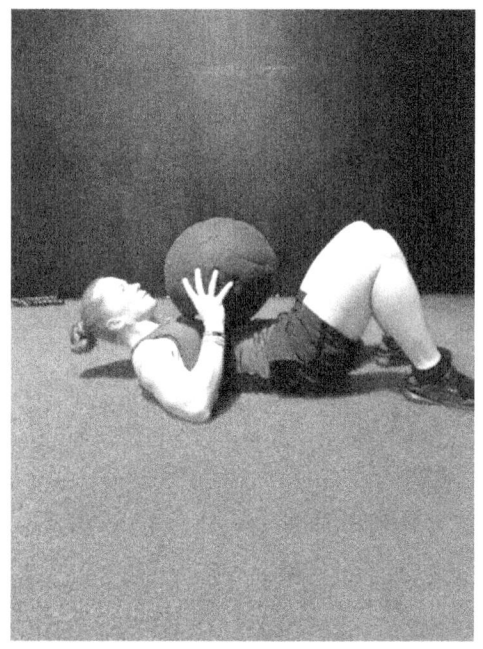

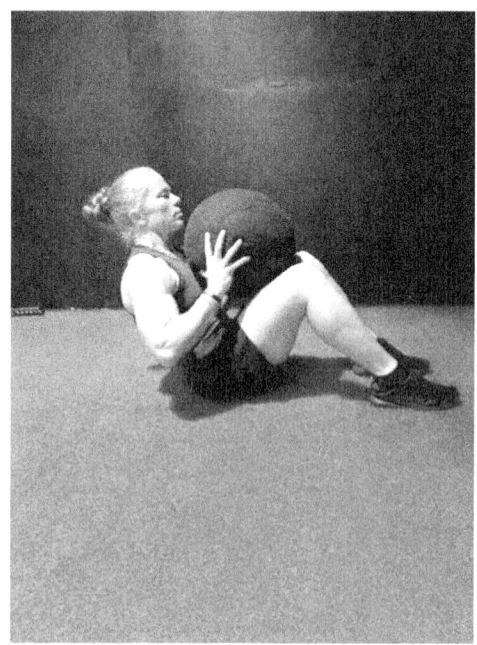

Sit-ups: Using resistance with abdominal exercises helps the abdominal muscle to grow against its tendons, which gives that definition needed for 6-pack abs. A medicine ball is a great way to provide resistance without the rigidity of a medicine ball or kettle bell.

Primary muscle: Abs

Secondary muscle: Lower back

Step:

1. Sit on the floor, with knees bent, feet flat on the ground, holding a medicine ball on your chest, under the chin.
2. Keeping your back straight, contract your abs, lifting your chest to your knees.
3. Lift far enough so that the medicine ball touches the knees, then lower yourself to the starting position in a controlled manner.
4. Repeat.

Keys: Keep the feet on the ground. Contract the abs throughout the movement, even when lowering, so that you're lowering at a controlled pace.

Medicine Ball Workout

LUNGE

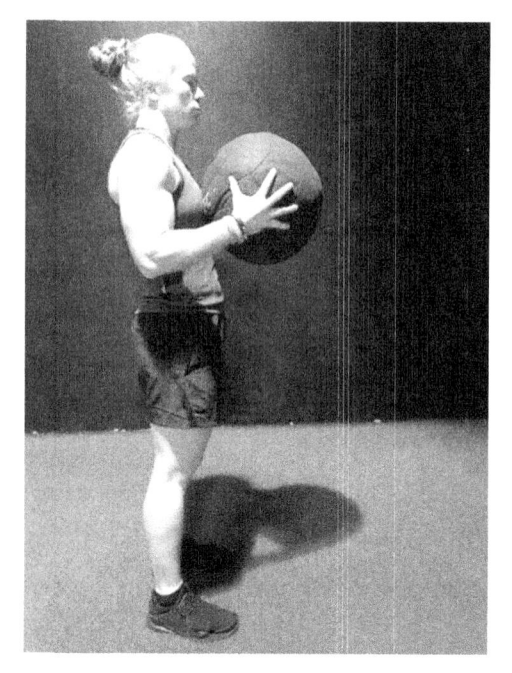

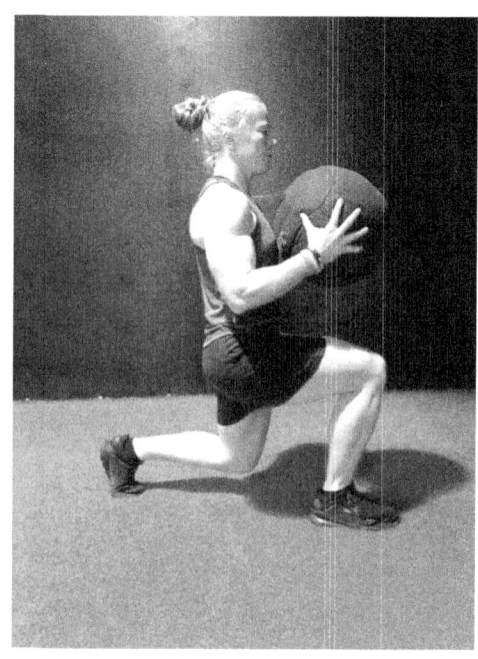

Lunge: The lunge is a foundational exercise to any resistance program. Adding a medicine ball increases the resistance and recruits secondary muscles in the arms to help support the weight.

Primary muscles: Quads, glutes

Secondary muscles: Hamstrings, biceps, shoulders

Steps:

1. Holding the medicine ball at chest level, step out with the right leg and plant the right foot on the floor.
2. Bending the right knee, lower body weight so that the knee angle is about 90 degrees (note: the knee and toe should be in line, and the knee shouldn't pass over the toe).
3. Press through the right leg, lifting yourself back to the standing position.
4. Repeat for the left leg.

Keys: Lunge out far enough so that the knee doesn't move past the toe. Keep the back straight during the lunge.

PUSHUPS

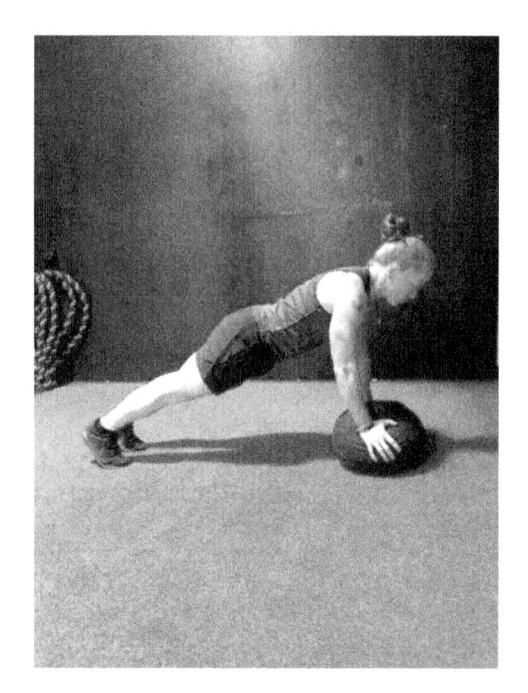

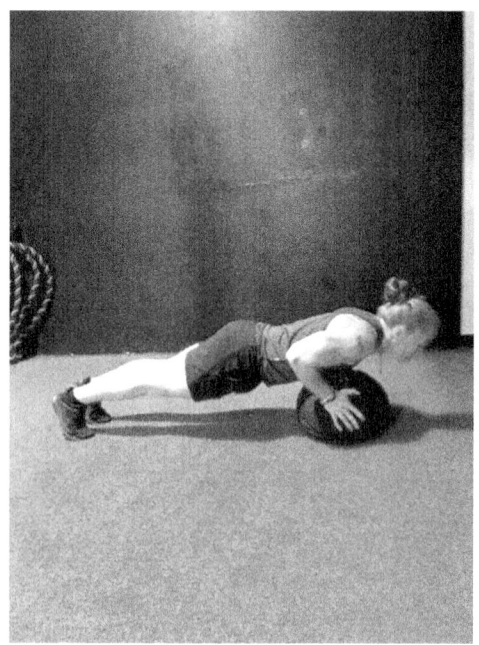

Pushups: Yet another foundational resistance exercise; just about everyone has done a pushup at some point. There are several variations of pushups you can do with a medicine ball. Performing the basic medicine ball pushup puts you on an unstable surface, recruiting stabilizer muscles.

Primary muscles: Chest, triceps

Secondary muscles: Shoulders, abs

Steps:

1. Position yourself with hands on the medicine ball in a plank position (prone).
2. Bending the elbows, lower your body until your chest touches the medicine ball, keeping your core tight and back straight.
3. Press up, still keeping the back straight and abs tight.
4. Repeat.

Keys: Keep the core tight, don't sway at the low back. Keep the back straight, don't arch.

OVERHEAD SQUAT

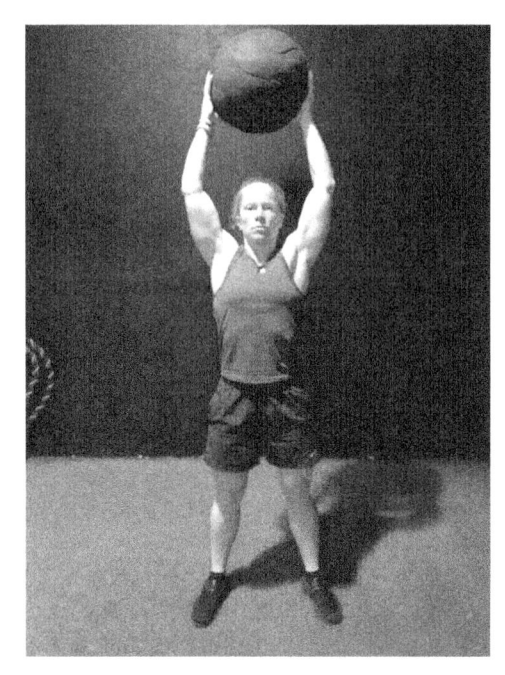

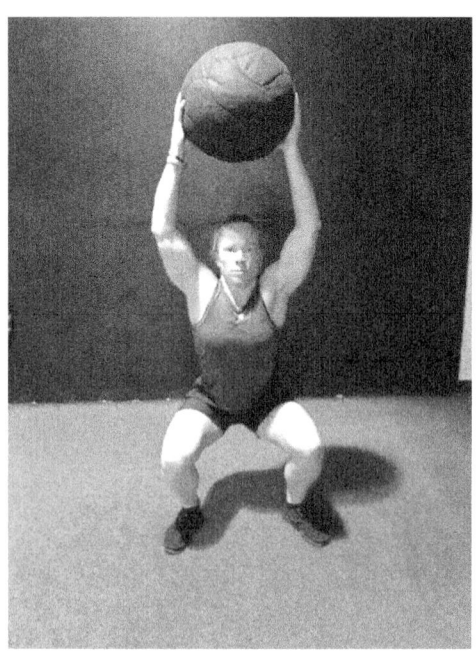

Overhead Squat: The overhead squat not only works the lower body, it hits the shoulders and core. You have to engage your core to keep the medicine ball stable overhead, and the load works to fatigue the shoulders.

Primary muscles: Quads, glutes

Secondary muscles: Shoulders, core

Steps:

1. Hold the medicine ball in both hands directly above your head, and stand with feet about shoulder-width apart (can be slightly wider).
2. Hinge at the hips, as if you're sitting in a chair, to initiate the squat, and bending the knees, squat down until your quads are parallel with the ground.
3. Engage the core to keep the ball steady and directly overhead.
4. Push through the heels and legs to raise yourself back into standing position with ball still overhead.
5. Repeat.

Keys: Hip hinge: bend at the hips first. Don't round or arch back. Knees track over the tops of the toes and not beyond the toes. Keep the medicine ball directly overhead and don't let the arms fall forward.

Medicine Ball Workout

CHEST PASS

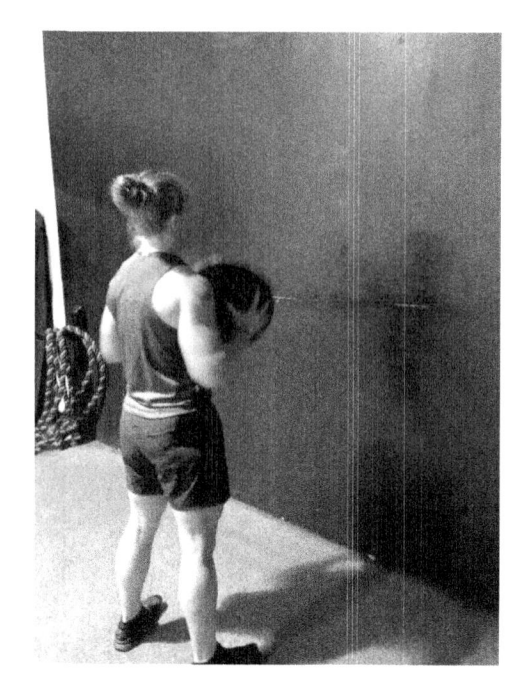

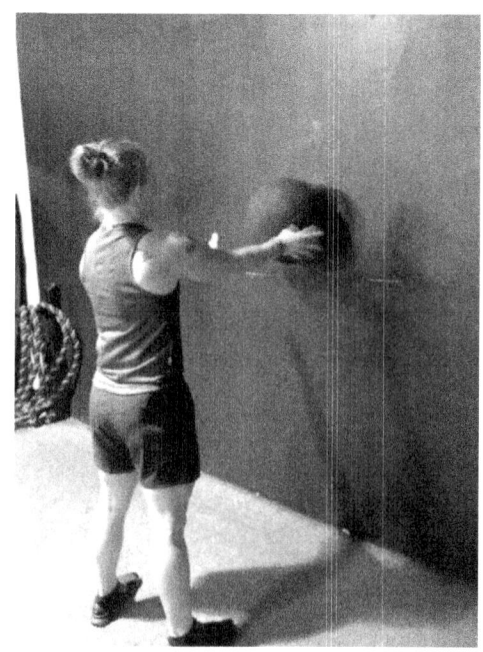

Chest pass: A simple upper body exercise, the chest pass engages the pectorals. It is an explosive exercise, so it can be used in a conditioning workout.

Primary muscles: Chest, triceps

Secondary muscles: Shoulders, abs

Steps:

1. Stand facing a wall, holding the medicine ball at chest height in both hands.

2. Pass the medicine ball from the chest straight into the wall, engaging the abs and pushing out with the arms as you do (to get more power, you can also incorporate a step forward).

3. Let the ball fall to the floor or catch it on the rebound, if you can.

4. Repeat.

Keys: Engage the abs to get power. The pass should be hard and explosive.

OVERHEAD PASS

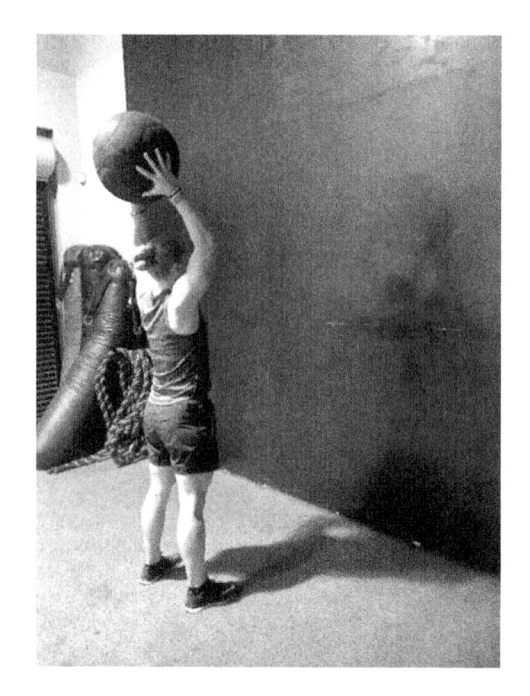

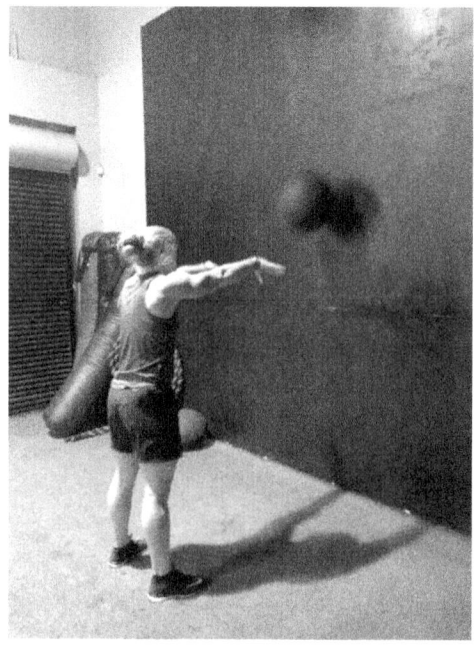

Overhead pass: Very similar to the chest pass, the overhead pass recruits the shoulders more than the chest, but is an explosive exercise as well.

Primary muscle: Shoulders

Secondary muscles: Chest, triceps, abs

Steps:

1. Stand facing a wall, holding the medicine ball in both hands overhead.
2. Pass the medicine ball from the overhead position into the wall, engaging the abs as you do (to get more power, incorporate a step forward).
3. Let the ball fall to the floor or catch it on the rebound.
4. Repeat.

Keys: Engage the abs to get power. Use power and explosiveness to throw the medicine ball into the wall.

OVERHEAD LATERAL BENDS

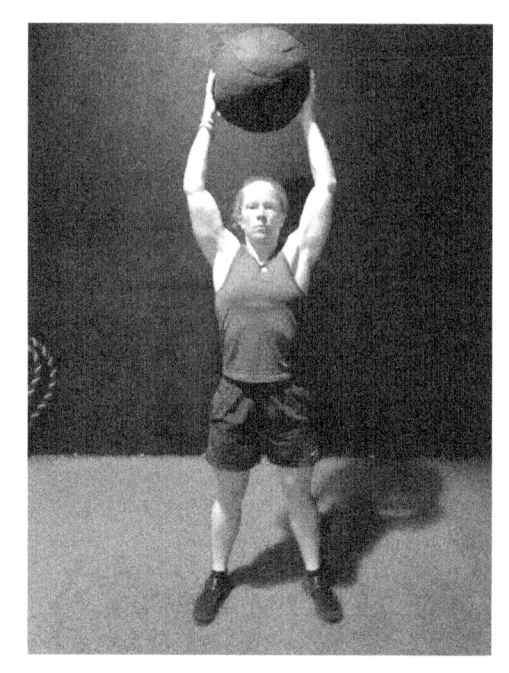

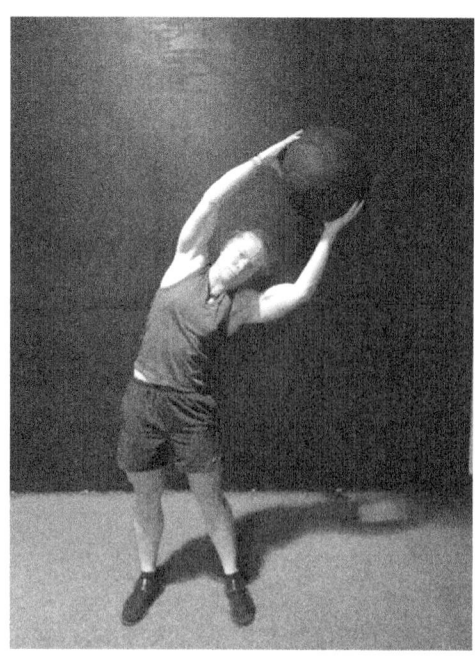

Overhead lateral bends: This is a simple core exercise that also recruits the shoulders to hold the load. Not only will it increase core strength, but it will also help range of motion and flexibility.

Primary muscles: Core (abs and obliques)

Secondary muscle: Shoulders

Steps:

1. Stand upright with the medicine ball directly overhead.
2. Push hips out to the right, bending the top of your body with the medicine ball to the left, stretching the right obliques and lats.
3. Engage the core to straighten your body.
4. Repeat with a bend to the right, and so on.

Keys: Keep the medicine ball over your head and don't let it sway. Keep your back straight and don't hunch over.

SHOULDER PRESS

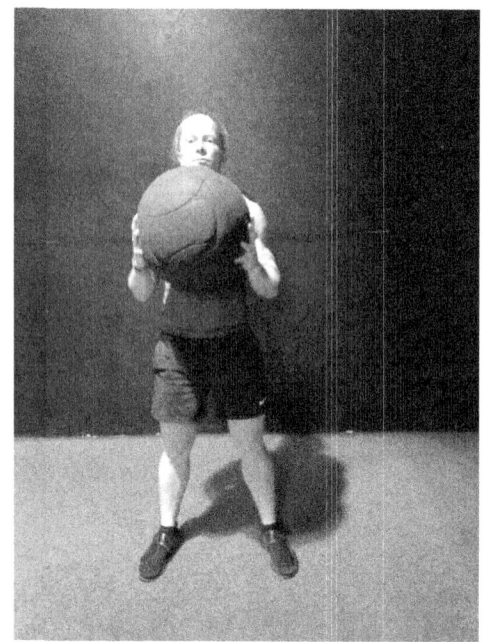

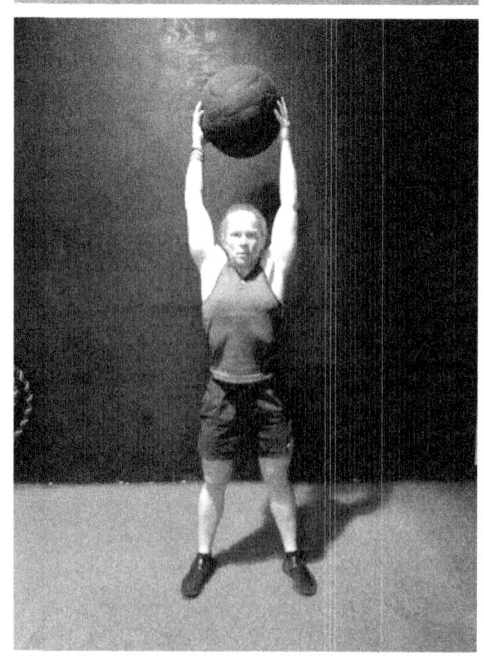

Shoulder press: The shoulder press is another standard resistance exercise, for which the medicine ball can be used as the load. It is a simple upper body exercise.

Primary muscles: Shoulders

Secondary muscles: Triceps

Steps:

1. From a standing position, hold the medicine ball at chest level, just under the chin.
2. Tuck chin back, and press medicine ball overhead (tuck the chin, so you can lift the load without hitting yourself).
3. As the medicine ball passes your head, push the head back through the arms and finish the movement with arms straight and medicine ball overhead.
4. Lower the medicine ball back to starting position and repeat.

Keys: Tucking the chin should be natural, but don't forget to push the head back through the arms (this gives you a little more power).

SUPERMANS

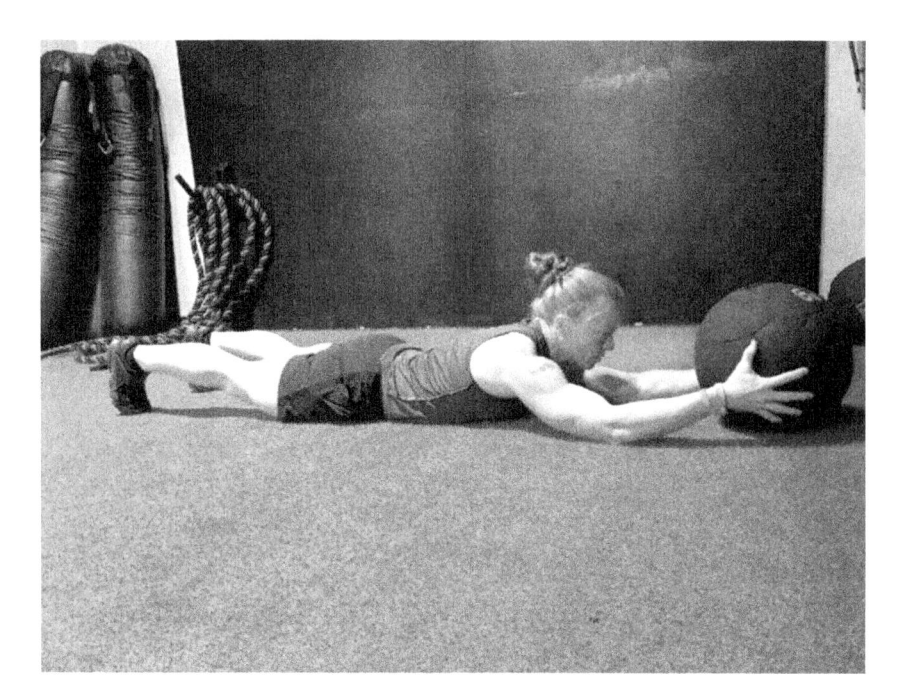

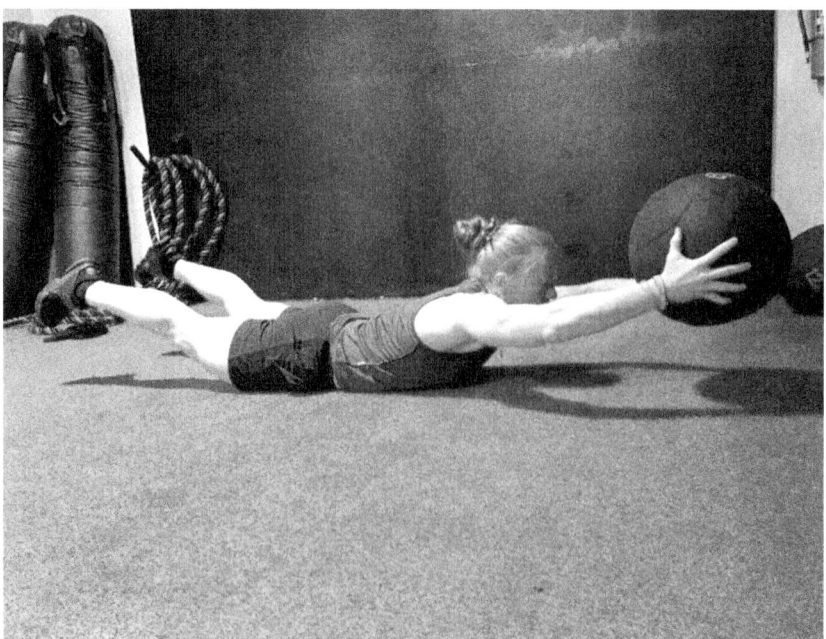

Superman: The Superman is a great core exercise. It's one of those exercises that looks easier than it is to perform. It works the lower and mid back (the often-neglected part of the core) and also the glutes.

Primary muscles: Back (lower and mid), glutes

Secondary muscles: Shoulders

Steps:

1. Lie prone on the floor, with arms extended overhead, holding the medicine ball in both hands.
2. Engage the lower and middle of the back to lift the arms and legs off the ground.
3. Squeeze the glutes and pinch the scapula back to lift further upward.
4. Return to prone position and repeat.

Keys: Be sure that the head is in a neutral position. To get as much lift as possible, concentrate on squeezing the glutes and pinching the scapula.

Chapter 6
Intermediate Medicine Ball Exercises

These intermediate exercises are a little more complex in movement than the simple exercises in the previous chapter. They work the body very hard. Advanced athletes as well as beginners will use these exercises.

Medicine Ball Workout

LUNGE WITH TWIST

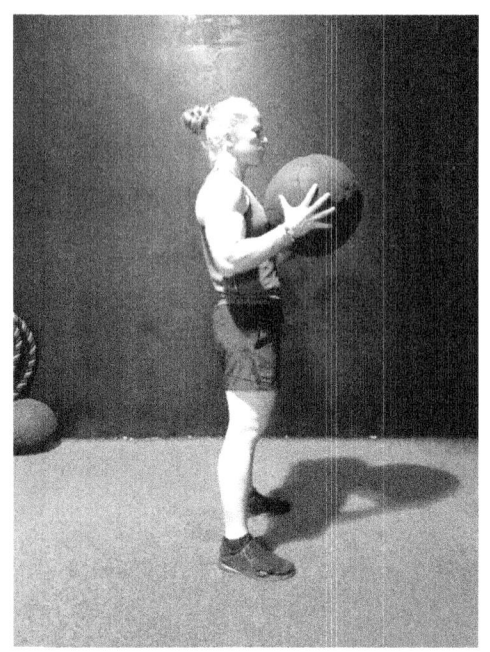

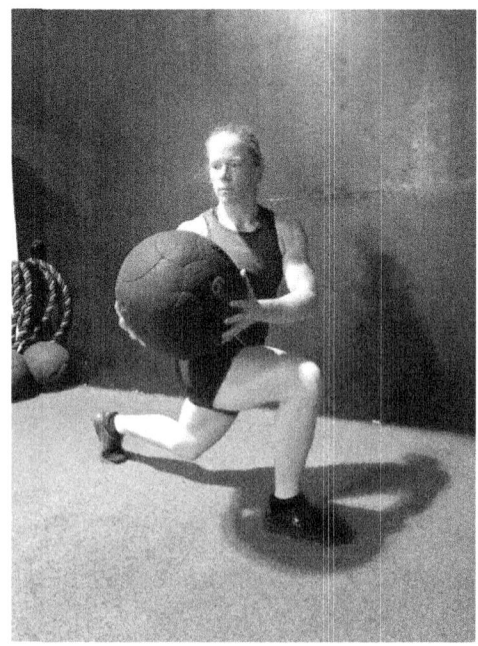

Lunge with twist: This is a variation of the lunge exercise. Adding a twist not only recruits core muscles, it also forces the stabilizer muscles to work harder.

Primary muscles: Quads, glutes, core (abs and obliques)

Secondary muscles: Hamstrings, biceps, shoulders

Steps:

1. Holding the medicine ball at chest level, step out with the right leg and plant the right foot on the floor.

2. Bending the right knee, lower body weight so that the knee angle is about 90 degrees (note: the knee and toe should be in line, and the knee shouldn't pass over the toe).

3. Twist with the medicine ball over the extended leg (to the same side as the leg, not away from it).

4. Press through the right leg lifting yourself back to the standing position.

5. Repeat for the left leg.

Keys: Lunge out far enough so that the knee doesn't move past the toe. Keep the back straight during the lunge and especially during the twist.

V-UPS

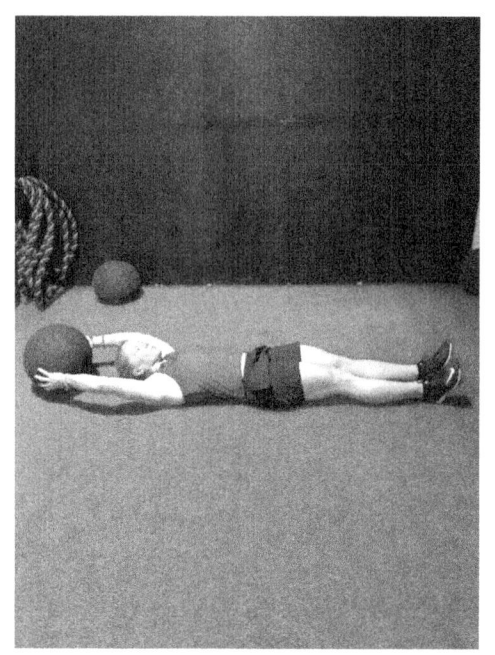

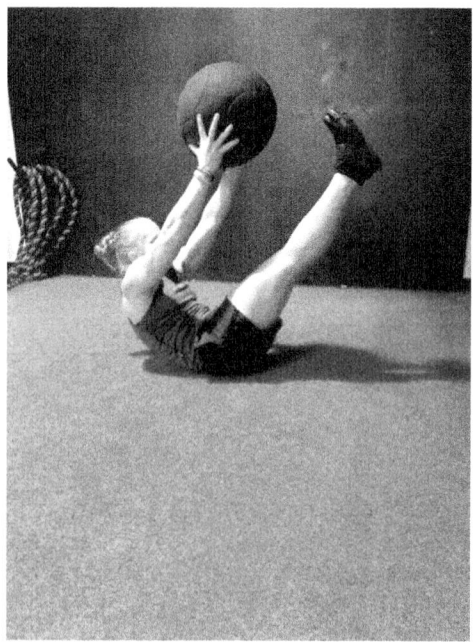

V-ups: This core exercise is a little more advanced than the sit-up or crunch. It requires movement with the upper and lower body and really forces you to engage your core.

Primary muscles: Core muscles

Secondary muscles: Shoulders

Steps:

1. Lie supine on the floor with arms overhead, holding the medicine ball in both hands.
2. Keeping arms and legs straight, lift both off the ground, engaging the core and bending the body at the hips, so that your body is in a V shape.
3. Bring the medicine ball forward and touch your toes.
4. Return medicine ball overhead while lowering your body back to supine position.
5. Repeat.

Keys: Keep your back straight and don't round. Try to keep the legs and arms straight through the entire movement.

Medicine Ball Workout

SIDE TOSS

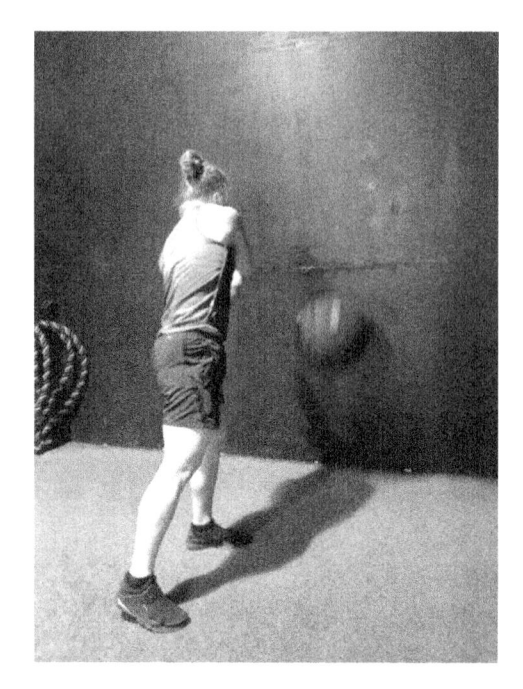

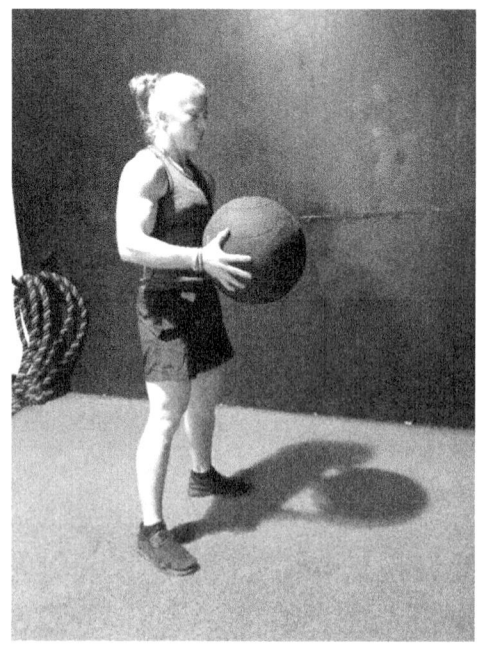

44

Side toss: Yet another core exercise, the side toss is similar to the chest pass, in that it requires explosive power. Not only does it work the core, but it helps with hip mobility.

Primary muscles: Core (abs and obliques)

Secondary muscles: Biceps, hip flexors

Steps:

1. Stand next to a wall (make sure the wall is on your right side), holding the medicine ball at stomach level, in both hands.
2. Rotate at the hips so that the medicine ball is on your left hip.
3. Engage the core and rotate the hips through, explosively, to the right, tossing the ball into the wall.
4. Let the ball fall to the ground or catch it on the rebound and return to the starting position.
5. Repeat for the other side.

Keys: Keep the back straight through the rotations. Use the arms to really slam the ball into the wall. Holding the ball underhand is the most effective.

Medicine Ball Workout

RUSSIAN TWIST

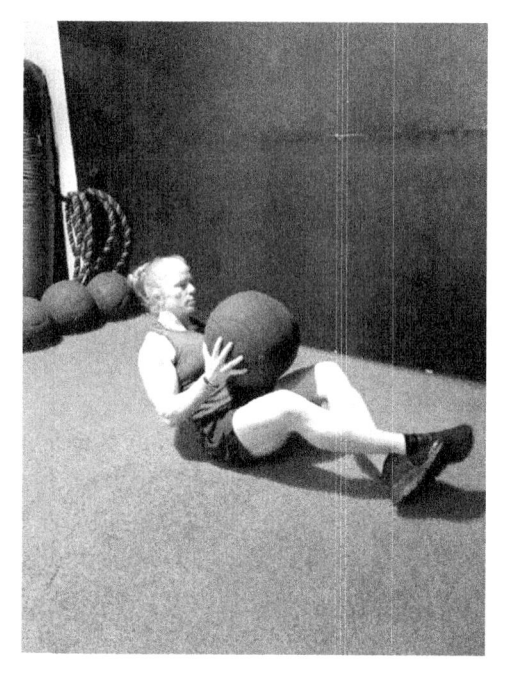

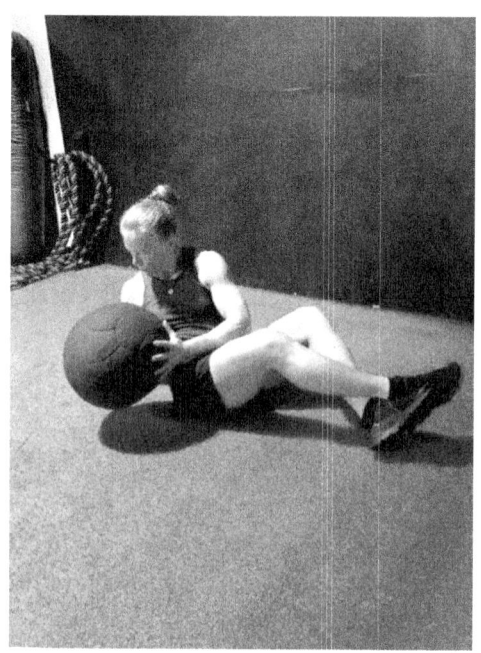

46

Russian twist: The Russian twist is a core exercise that can be done with or without resistance. Adding resistance makes it more difficult and really works the obliques.

Primary muscles: Core (abs and obliques)

Secondary muscles: Biceps

Steps:

1. Start sitting on the floor with knees bent and your feet off the ground. Hold the medicine ball in both hands at your stomach.

2. Engage the core and rotate the medicine ball down to the left side, touching the floor beside your hip.

3. Return to the starting position and then rotate to the right side, touching the medicine ball to the floor beside the right hip.

4. Repeat.

Keys: Keep the back straight. Don't let the feet touch the ground. Keep your elbows locked in to avoid too much movement in the arms (it's about twisting your core, not placing the medicine ball to your side with your arms).

Medicine Ball Workout

WOODCHOPPER

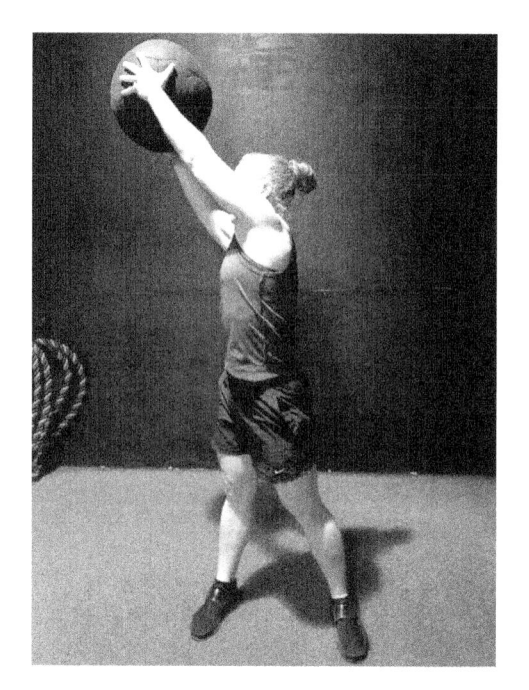

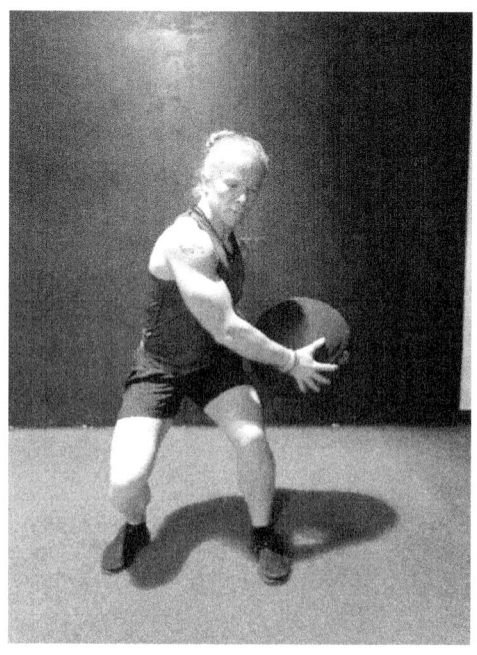

Woodchopper: The woodchopper is a total body exercise, recruiting the legs, upper body and core. It is good for mobility as well as building a strong core.

Primary muscles: Core (abs, obliques, lower back)

Secondary muscles: Quads, shoulders

Steps:

1. Start with feet about shoulder-width apart, holding the medicine ball in both hands.
2. Raise medicine ball over the left shoulder, rotating the hips to the left.
3. In a chopping motion, bring the medicine ball across the body and alongside the right knee, rotating the hips and bending slightly at the knees.
4. Push through the legs, rotate the hips and return the medicine ball to the position above the left shoulder.
5. Repeat and then switch sides.

Keys: Focus on the rotation of the torso. Keep back straight and don't hunch over. Move with force but also with control.

HALO SLAM

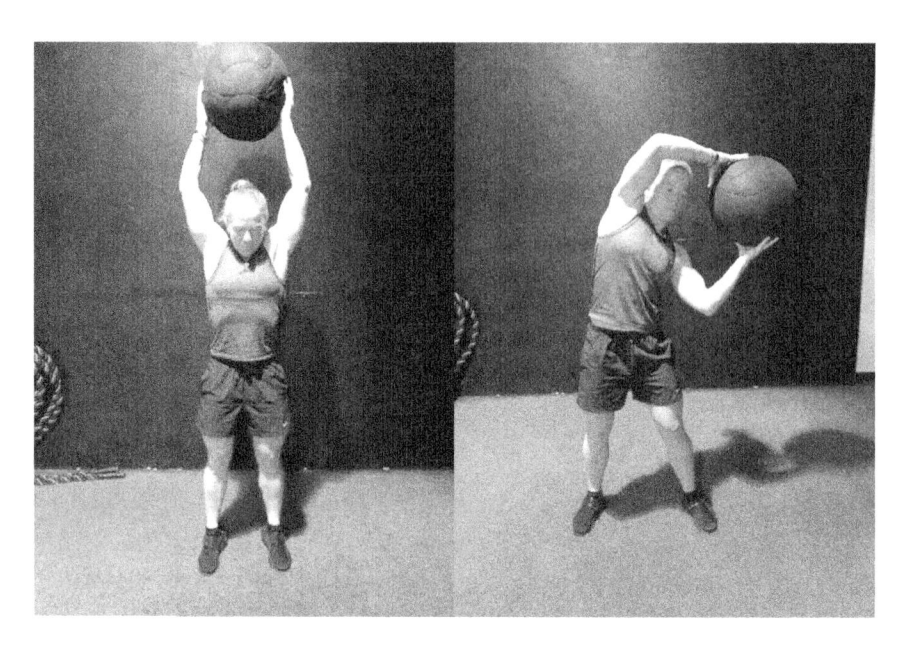

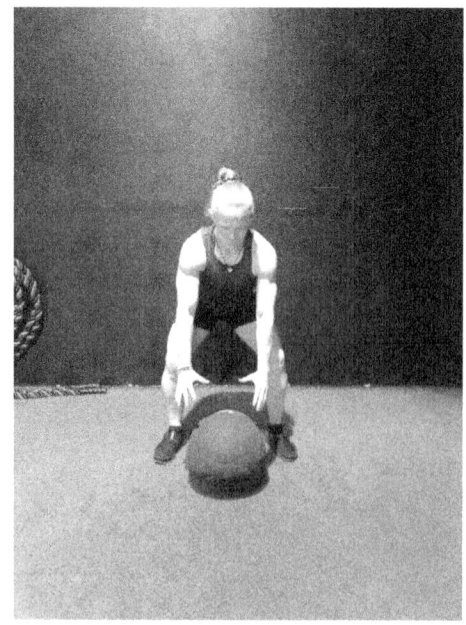

Halo slam: The halo slam is a variation of the basic slam. Performing the slam in a halo motion works shoulder mobility and better engages the core.

Primary muscles: Lats, shoulders, abs

Secondary muscles: Legs

Steps:

1. Start standing, holding the medicine ball in both hands.
2. Bring the medicine ball overhead in a half circle (halo) motion to the right.
3. Forcefully throw the medicine ball to the ground, in front of your feet, contracting the abs and bringing the arms through, ending with the knees slightly bent.
4. If possible, catch the ball on the bounce. Otherwise, pick the medicine ball up from the ground.
5. Repeat, bringing the medicine ball in a halo motion around to the left.

Keys: Start the slam motion fully extended. Slam the ball forcefully into the ground, contracting the abs.

STAGGERED PUSHUP

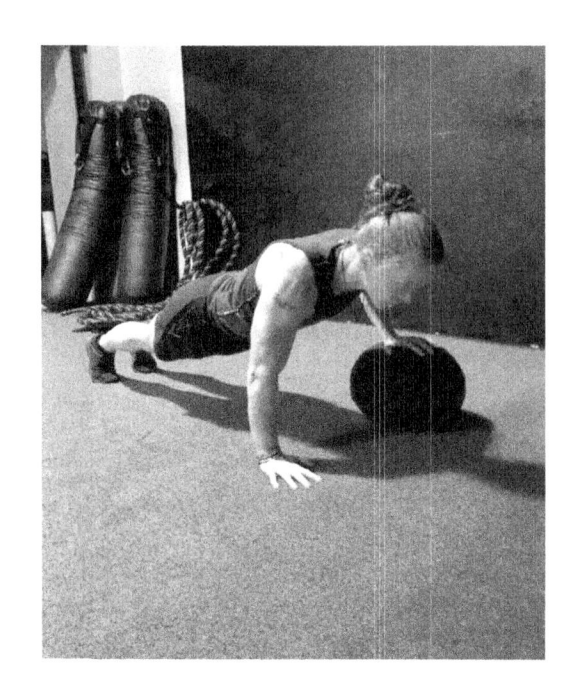

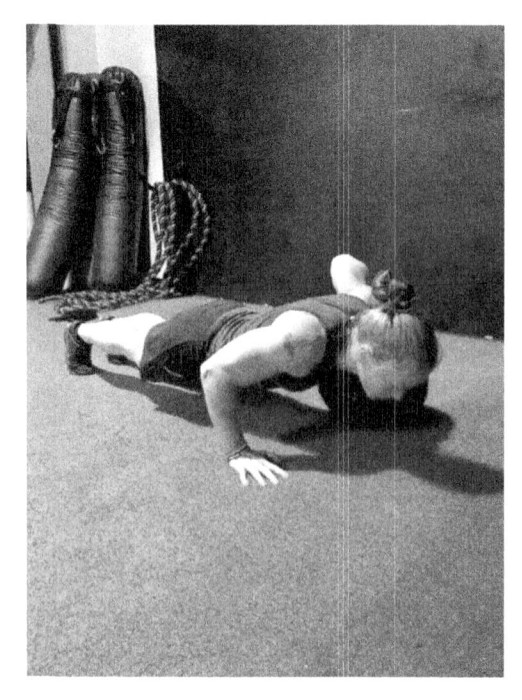

Staggered pushup: A variation of the standard pushup, the staggered pushup takes the medicine ball pushup to the next level. It is an upper body exercise, but it also recruits the core for stability purposes.

Primary muscles: Chest, triceps

Secondary muscles: Shoulders, abs

Steps:

1. Position yourself with one hand on the medicine ball in a plank position (prone) and one hand on the floor.
2. Bending the elbows, lower your body until your chest is even with the medicine ball, keeping your core tight and back straight.
3. Press up, still keeping the back straight and abs tight.
4. Roll the ball to the hand that was on the ground and place that hand on the medicine ball and the other on the floor
5. Repeat.

Keys: Keep the core tight, don't sway at the low back. Keep the back straight, don't arch.

OVERHEAD WALKING LUNGE

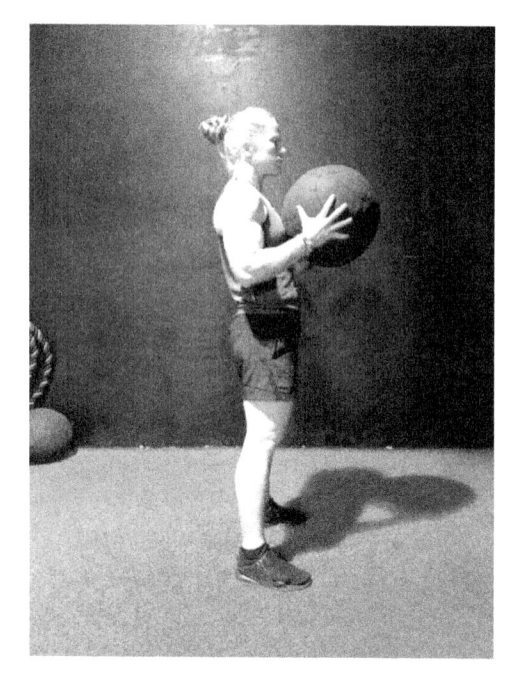

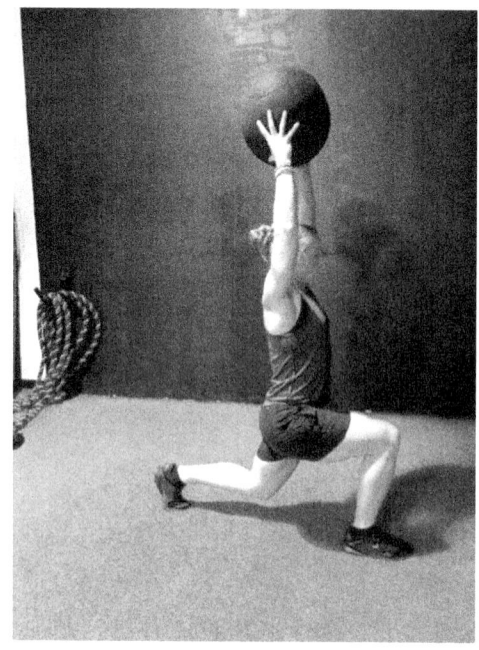

Overhead walking lunge: Yet another lunge variation, this exercise takes the principles of the overhead squat (core stability and shoulder mobility) and puts them in lunge form. Walking out the lunge will also test your balance.

Primary muscles: Quads, glutes

Secondary muscles: Hamstrings, shoulders, core

Steps:

1. Start standing, holding the medicine ball in both hands overhead.
2. Step out with the right leg and plant the right foot on the floor.
3. Bending the right knee, lower body weight so that the knee angle is about 90 degrees (note: the knee and toe should be in line, and the knee shouldn't pass over the toe), keeping the medicine ball overhead.
4. Pushing through the right leg, bring the left leg back in line with the right in a standing position.
5. Next, lunge out with the left leg.
6. Repeat, walking forward with each leg.

Keys: Keep the arms straight overhead and don't let them fall forward. Keep the back straight and the core tight.

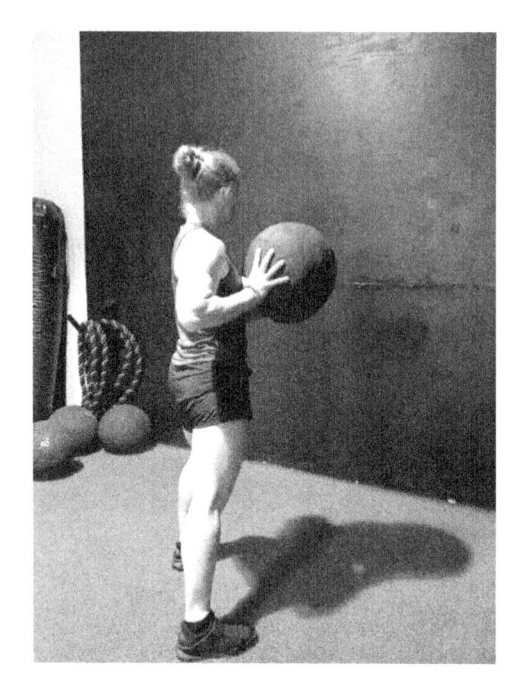

SINGLE ARM CHEST PASS

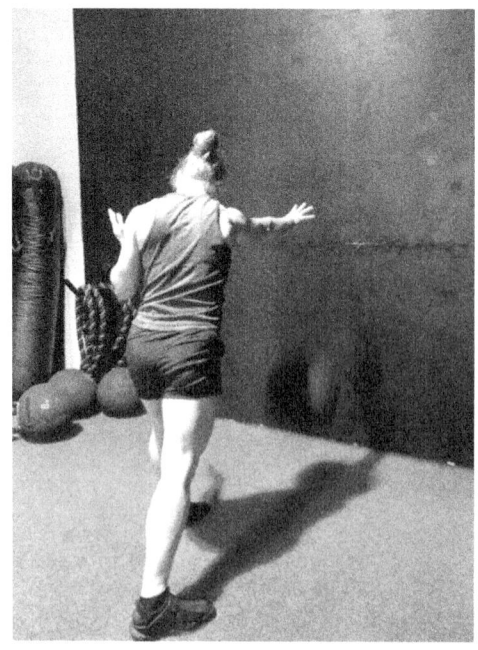

Single arm chest pass: This is a variation of the chest pass, in which you'll only use one arm to slam the medicine ball, from the chest, into the wall.

Primary muscles: Chest, obliques

Secondary muscles: Triceps

Steps:

1. Stand facing a wall and hold the medicine ball to the right of your chest, with your right hand behind the ball and left hand to the side.

2. Step forward with the right leg and push with the right arm, slamming the ball into the wall.

3. Let the medicine ball drop to the floor or catch it on the rebound.

4. Switch arms and repeat.

Keys: Pass the medicine ball forcefully into the wall. Keep the core engaged. Rotate the hips through on the passing motion.

THRUSTER

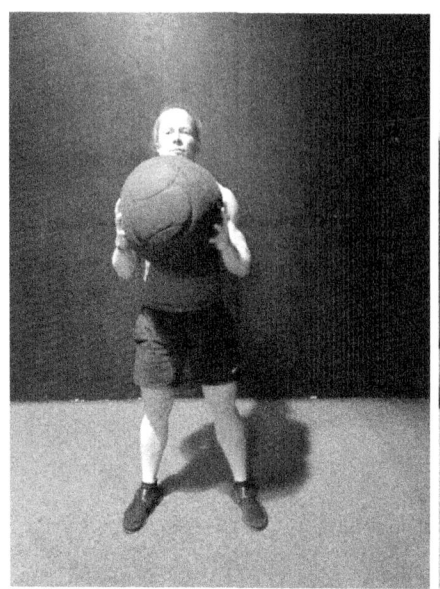

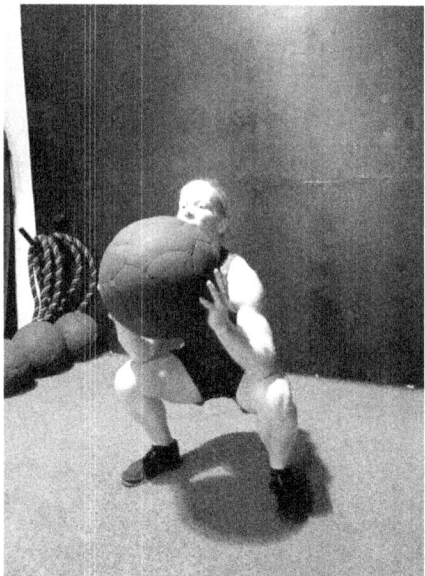

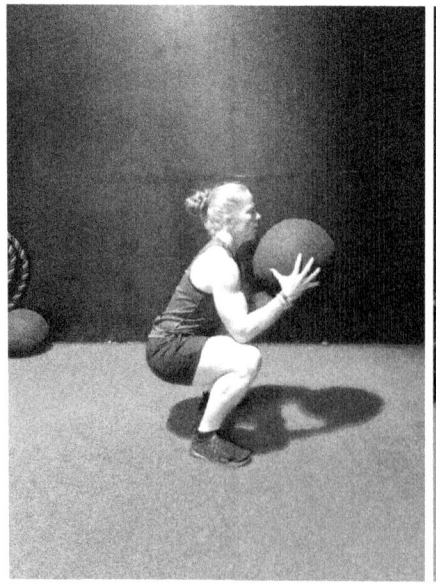

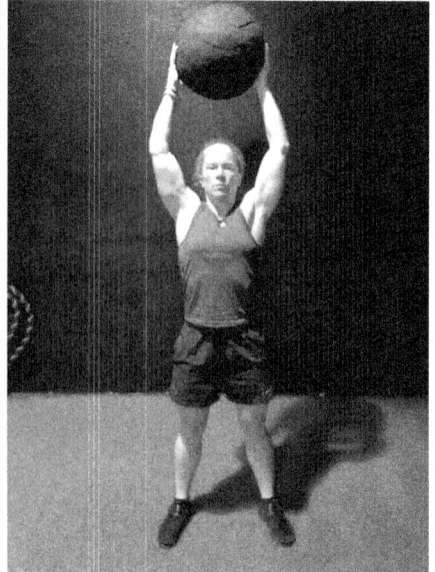

Thruster: The thruster is a combination of a squat and a shoulder press. Combining these two exercises makes the thruster very effective in training both the upper and lower body.

Primary muscles: Quads, glutes, shoulders

Secondary muscles: Core

Steps:

1. Start with feet slightly wider than shoulder-width apart, holding the medicine ball in both hands at chest level.
2. Hinge at the hips and bend at the knees, squatting low enough to touch your elbows to your knees.
3. Push through the legs to raise yourself.
4. As you're finishing the upward motion, press the medicine ball overhead, tucking the chin as it passes your head and then pushing your head through as you press the medicine ball.
5. Lower the ball back to chest level and repeat.

Keys: Keep the back straight. Don't round and don't arch the back. Engage the core as you raise your body and press the ball. Use the chin tuck and send the head through to thrust the medicine ball upward.

Chapter 7
Complex Medicine Ball Exercises

These complex medicine ball exercises will have multiple movements and often combine two simple exercises. Combining the exercises works on your endurance as well as your strength. There's also some explosive movements worked in which are called plyometrics. These will help with your power.

Just because they're complex does not mean there better than the other exercises; they just take a different approach. We won't go into the different types of muscle fibers in this book, but you have several different muscle fibers that need to be trained in different ways. These complex movements are great for training fibers that work on your muscular endurance.

WALL BALL

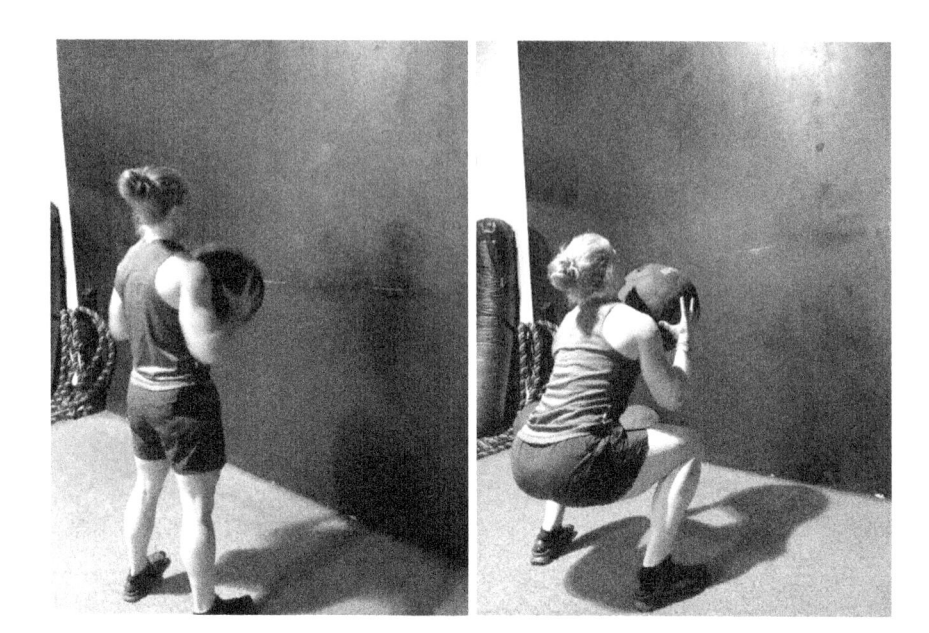

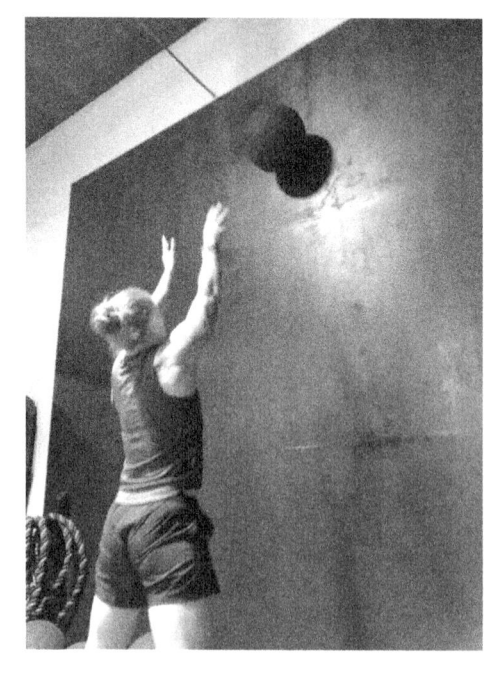

Wall ball: This is a complex exercise that takes the thruster to the next level. It engages the lower body, core and shoulders through the motion, and it tests your hand-eye coordination.

Primary muscles: Quads, glutes, shoulders

Secondary muscles: Core

Steps:

1. Start facing a wall, with feet slightly wider than shoulder-width apart, holding the medicine ball in both hands at chest level.

2. Hinge at the hips and bend at the knees, squatting low enough to touch your elbows to your knees.

3. Push through the legs to raise yourself in an explosive motion.

4. As you're coming up out of the squat position, thrust the medicine ball upward, tossing it high up on the wall.

5. Catch the ball as it's falling, and let the momentum take you back into the squat position.

6. Repeat the squat and throw.

Keys: Keep the back straight and don't hunch. The upward motion is an explosive one, as is the toss high on the wall. This should be a fluid motion, from the catch back into the squat.

BURPEE SLAMS

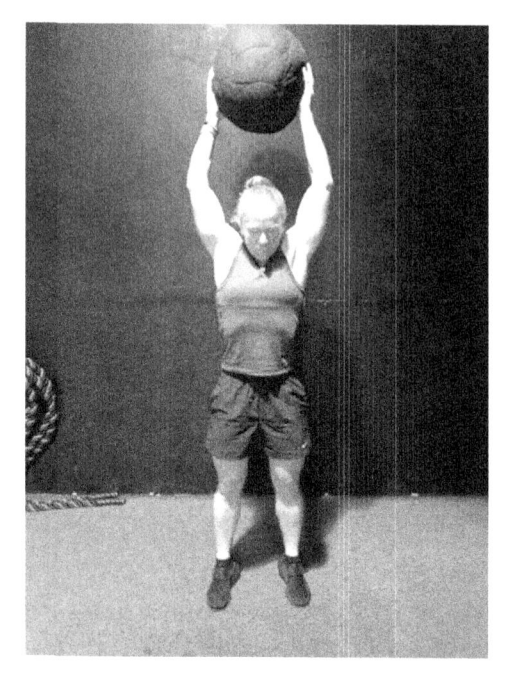

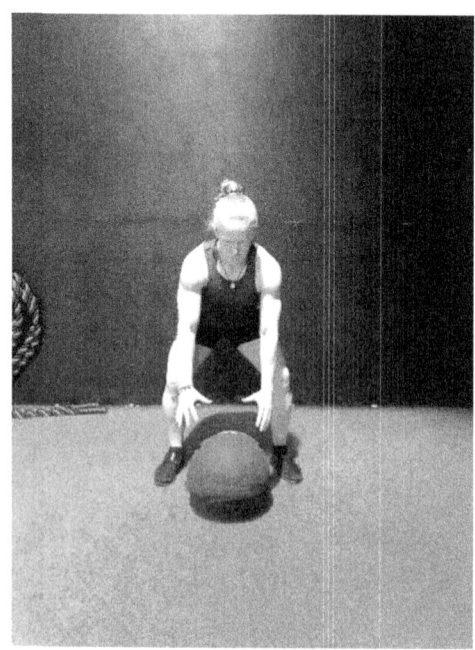

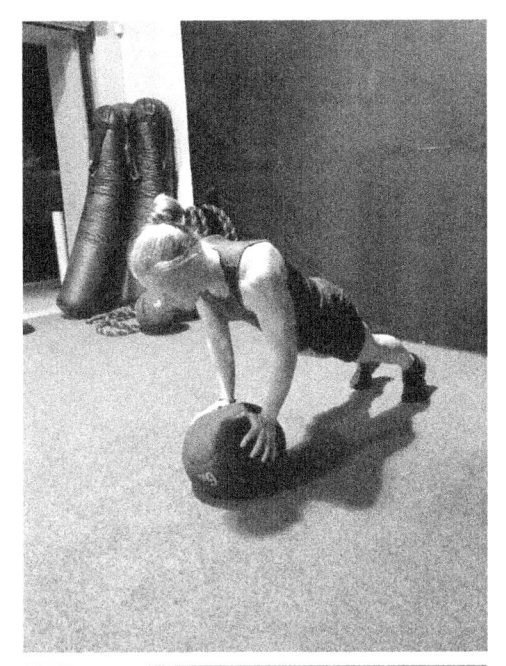

Complex Medicine Ball Exercises

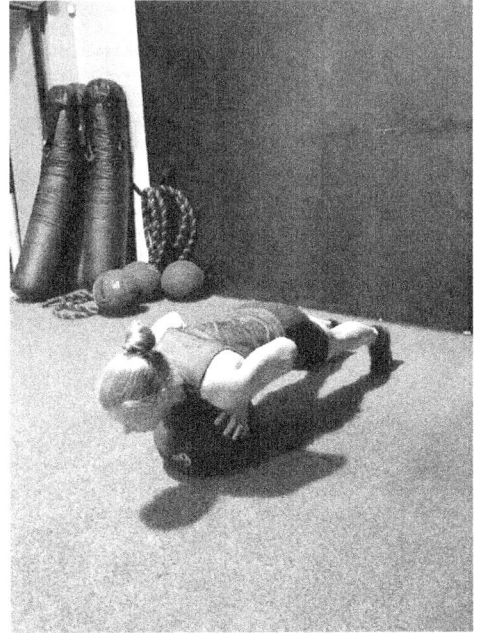

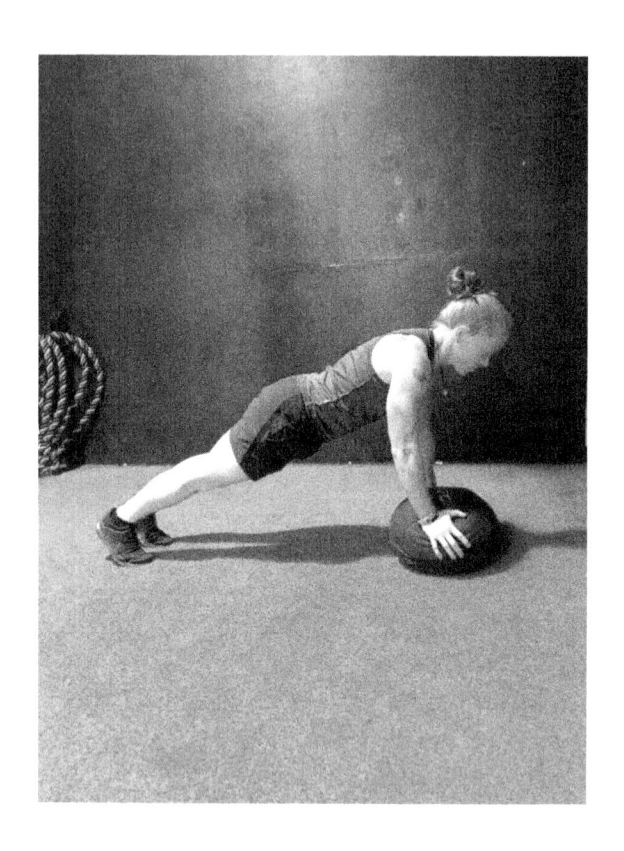

Medicine Ball Workout

Burpee slams: A variation on the medicine ball slam, the burpee slam incorporates a burpee. A burpee by itself is a great bodyweight exercise. Combining the slam and burpee is a great way to work the whole body with an explosive and functional movement.

Primary muscles: Lats, legs, chest

Secondary muscles: Shoulders, core

Steps:

1. Stand with feet shoulder-width apart, holding the medicine ball overhead.
2. Forcefully throw the medicine ball to the ground, in front of your feet, contracting the abs and bringing the arms through, ending with the knees slightly bent.
3. Drop your body to the ground, landing your hands on the medicine ball, and then extend your feet so that you're in a plank position.
4. Perform a pushup on the medicine ball, and then hop your feet to your chest, close to the medicine ball.
5. Grasping the medicine ball, pick yourself and it up into a standing position.
6. Jump into the air with the medicine ball overhead.
7. On the way down, repeat, performing the slam.

Keys: The slam should be forceful. Keep the core tight in the slam as well as in the plank position and through the pushup. The drop to the ground and extension of the feet should be done quickly, yet fluidly.

IN AND OUT PUSHUPS

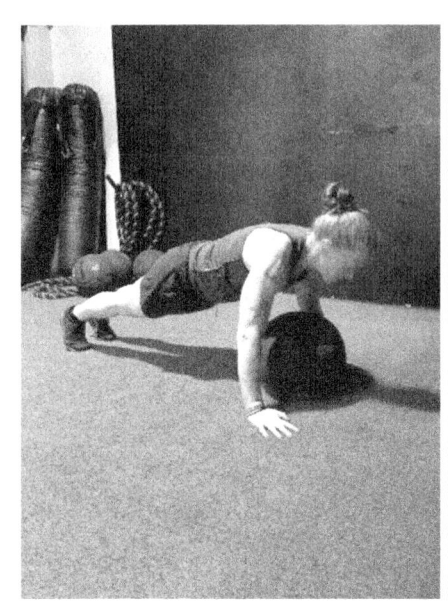

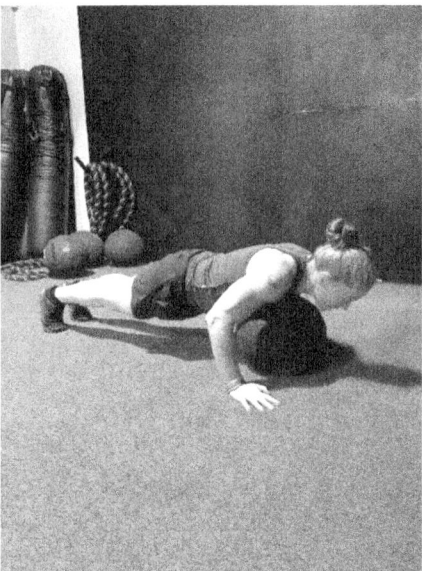

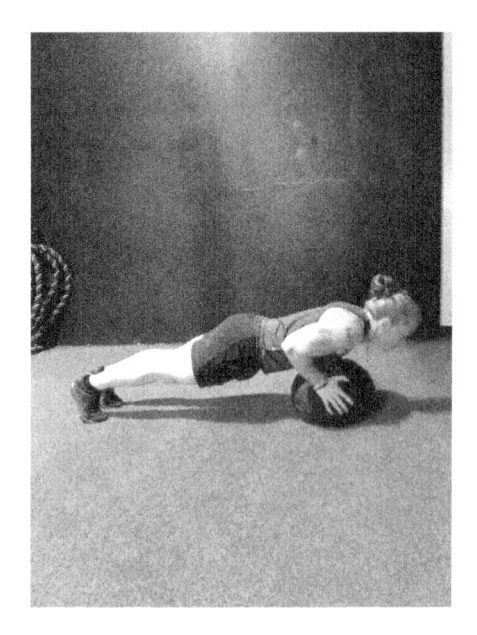

In and out pushups: This is an explosive pushup variation on the medicine ball. It requires great power to perform it correctly and will test your upper body strength.

Primary muscles: Chest, core

Secondary muscles: Triceps, shoulders

Steps:

1. Position yourself with hands on the medicine ball in a plank position (prone).
2. Bending the elbows, lower your body until your chest touches the medicine ball, keeping your core tight and back straight.
3. Press up through the chest forcefully enough to lift your hands from the medicine ball and switch their position to outside the medicine ball.
4. Catching yourself in a wide-arm position outside the medicine ball, lower your body until it touches the medicine ball.
5. In another explosive press upward through the chest, catch yourself in the original starting position.
6. Repeat.

Keys: With each press, you are using enough force so that you can lift your hands and reposition them. Keep the back straight and core engaged. Don't sway or arch the back.

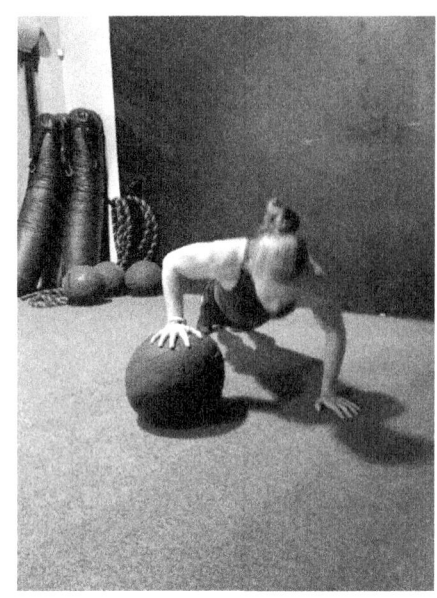

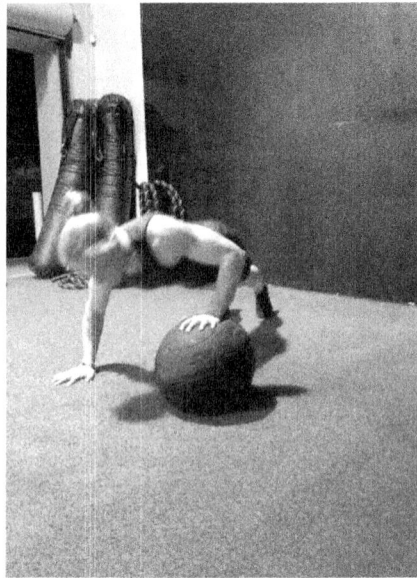

ALTERNATING PUSHUPS

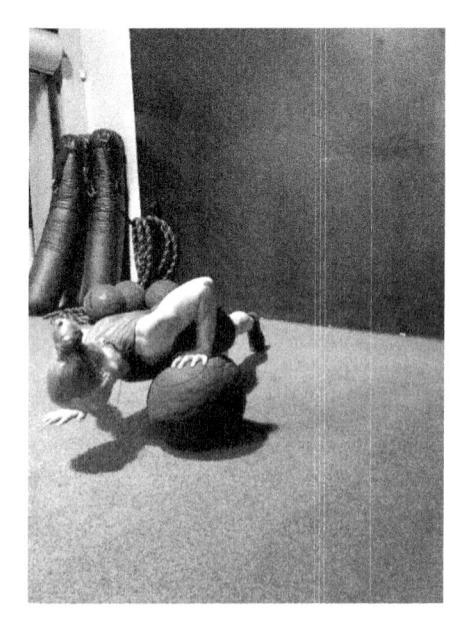

Alternating pushups: This pushup variation will take the staggered push-up to the next level. This one will also test your upper body strength and force you to engage your core.

Primary muscles: Chest, core

Secondary muscles: Triceps, shoulders

Steps:

1. Position yourself with the right hand on the medicine ball in a plank position (prone) and with the left hand on the floor.

2. Bending the elbows, lower your body until your chest is even with the medicine ball, keeping your core tight and your back straight.

3. Press up forcefully and explode to the right side, changing your hand placement, so that you catch yourself with the left hand on the medicine ball and the right hand on the floor.

4. Repeat for the left side, changing hand placement at every explosive push upward.

Keys: With each press you are using enough force so that you can lift your hands and reposition them. Keep the back straight and core engaged. Don't sway or arch the back.

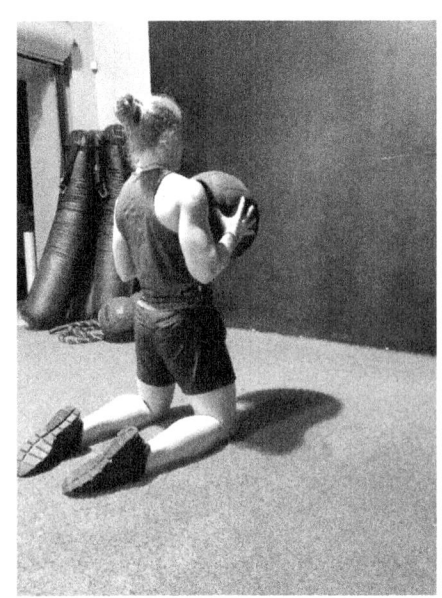

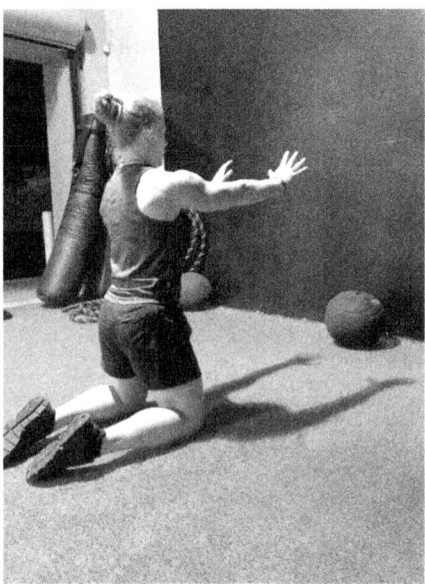

CHEST PASS TO PUSHUPS

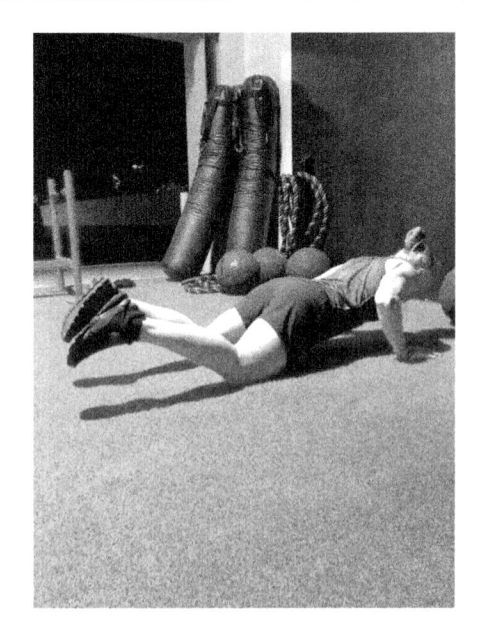

Chest pass to pushups: This exercise combines pushups and the medicine ball chest pass into a complex exercise that works the upper body hard. You'll also need good core strength to do this one.

Primary muscles: Chest, core

Secondary muscles: Triceps, shoulders

Steps:

1. Start on your knees, facing a wall, with the medicine ball in both hands at chest level.
2. Push through the chest and throw the medicine ball into the wall.
3. Let the force of the push bring you down to the floor and catch yourself with your hands, knees still bent.
4. Perform an explosive pushup on your knees to return to the start position.
5. Retrieve the medicine ball in front of you and repeat.

Keys: You should be close enough to the wall so that the medicine ball rebounds within arms' reach, so that you don't have to get up to retrieve it. Both the pass and the pushup are explosive movements. Keep the back straight and core engaged.

BURPEE WALL BALL

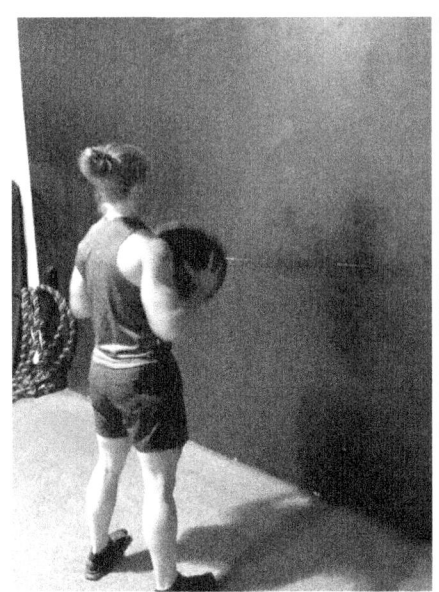

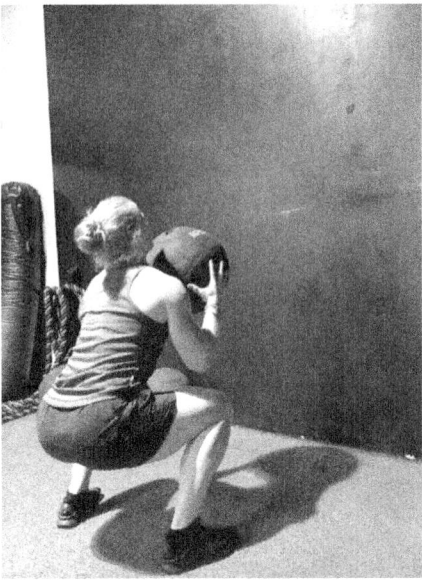

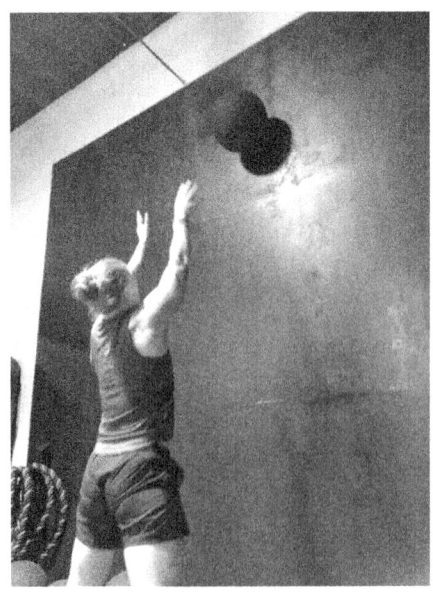

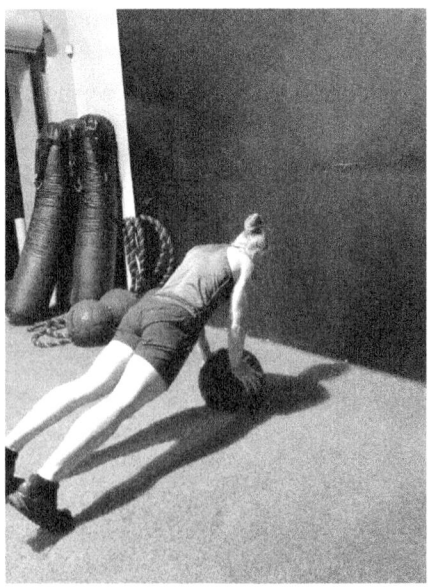

Burpee wall ball: Like many of the other complex exercises, the burpee wall ball combines a few different movements. This exercise by itself is exhausting and will test your entire body, as well as your hand-eye coordination.

Primary muscles: Quads, glutes, chest, shoulders

Secondary muscles: Triceps, core

Steps:

1. Start facing a wall, with feet slightly wider than shoulder-width apart, holding the medicine ball in both hands at chest level.
2. Hinge at the hips and bend at the knees, squatting low enough to touch your elbows to your knees.
3. Push through the legs to raise yourself in an explosive motion.
4. As you're coming up out of the squat position, thrust the medicine ball upward, tossing it high up on the wall.
5. Catch the ball as it's falling and drop it to the ground.
6. Drop your body to the ground, landing your hands on the medicine ball and then extend your feet so that you're in a plank position.
7. Perform a pushup on the medicine ball, and then hop your feet to your chest, close to the medicine ball.
8. Grasping the medicine ball, pick yourself and it up into a standing position.
9. Repeat.

Keys: Basically, you're performing a wall ball and then a burpee on the medicine ball. Keep the back straight through the entire movement. Keep the core engaged.

LUNGE SLAM

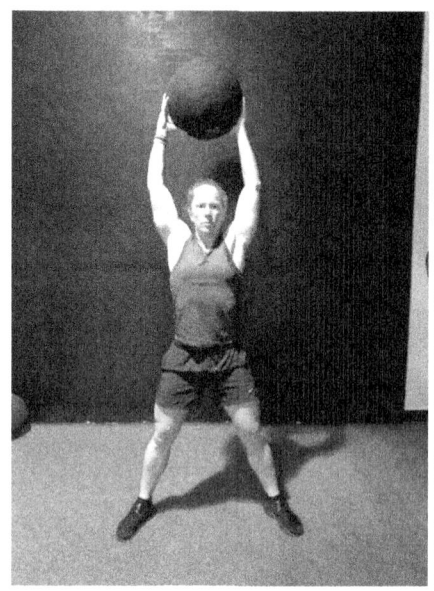

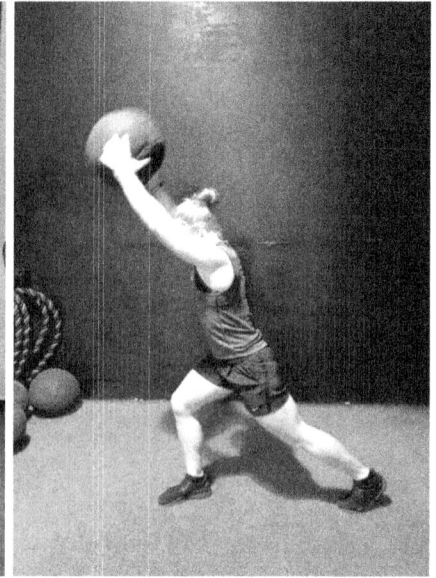

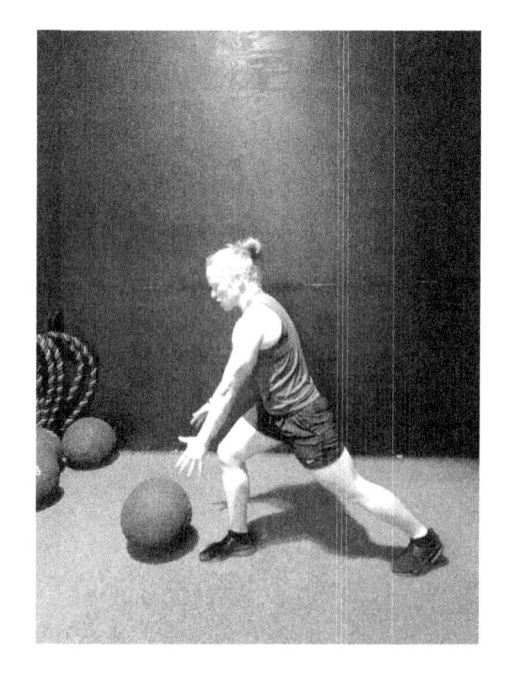

Lunge slam: This is another variation on the medicine ball slam. The lunge slam combines a lunge and a medicine ball slam. Not only will you recruit both upper and lower body muscles, you will also work on your balance and range of motion.

Primary muscles: Glutes, quads, shoulders

Secondary muscles: Hamstrings, core

Steps:

1. Start in a wide stance, with the medicine ball overhead.
2. Turn your feet and body to the right and slam the ball down in front of your right foot, bringing your body down into a lunge position.
3. Catch the ball on the rebound, or pick it up, and lift it back overhead, turning your body to face forward again.
4. Turn your feet and body to the left in a fluid motion and repeat the slam and lunge on the left side.
5. Alternate sides.

Keys: Keep the back straight and don't hunch over in the slam. Concentrate on the hip rotation with each movement. Keep the core engaged on the slam. This should be a fluid movement from slam to slam.

SPRINTER START CHEST PASS

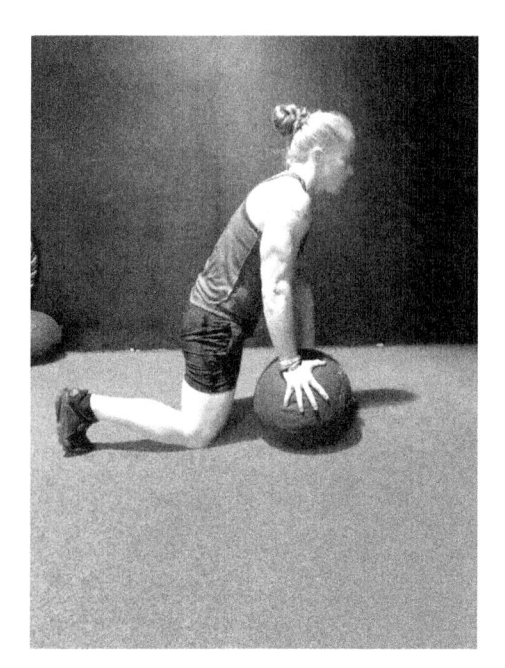

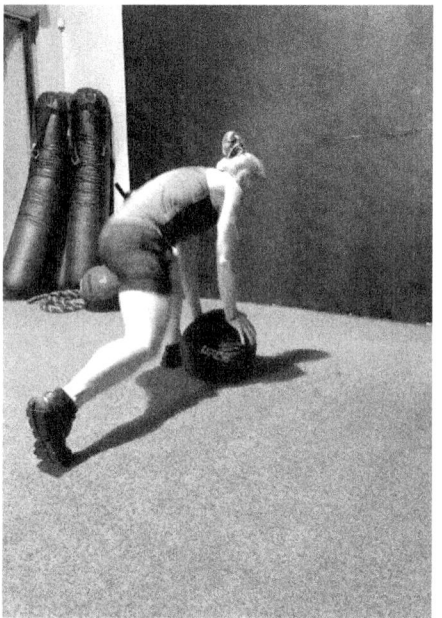

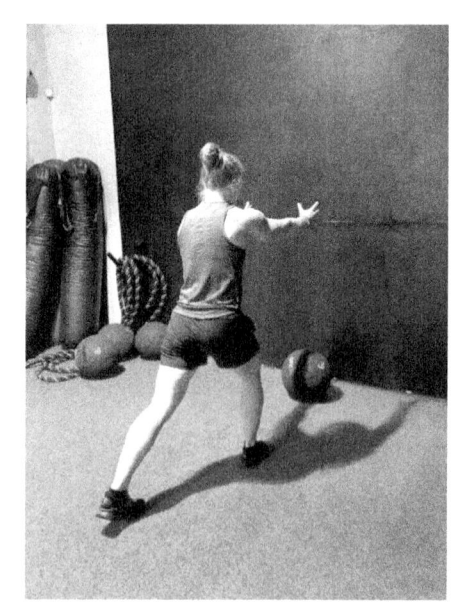

Sprinter start chest pass: This is an explosive exercise that is used by athletes to improve their power from a sprint position. It works the lower body as well as the chest and core.

Primary muscles: Glutes, quads, chest

Secondary muscles: Hamstrings, core

Steps:

1. Start in a lunge position, with the right knee up and left knee on the floor, in front of a wall.

2. Position the medicine ball in front of the left knee and grasp it with both hands, bending slightly.

3. Like a sprinter, push through the right leg and lift the left leg in a sprint motion forward, picking up the medicine ball in the motion.

4. As you're moving forward with the left leg, bring the medicine ball up and press through the chest, throwing the ball into the wall.

5. Retrieve the medicine ball and reposition with the left leg up and right knee on the floor.

6. Repeat.

Keys: Picture yourself as a sprinter in the blocks about to start a race. The movement forward should mimic a sprint start. The chest pass is explosive and forceful. Engage the core throughout the movement.

Medicine Ball Workout

SQUAT ROCKERS

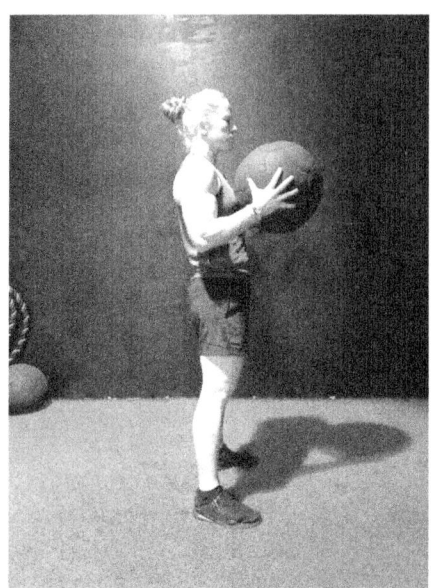

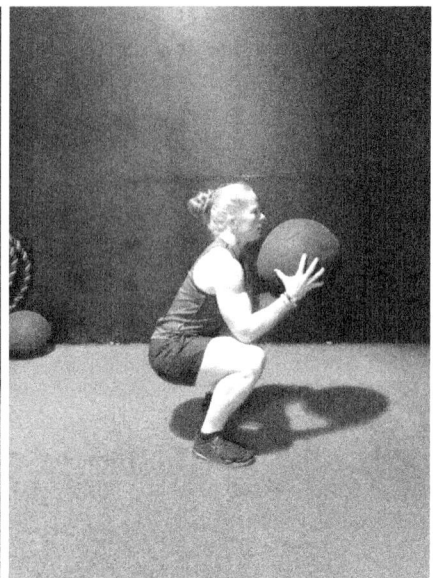

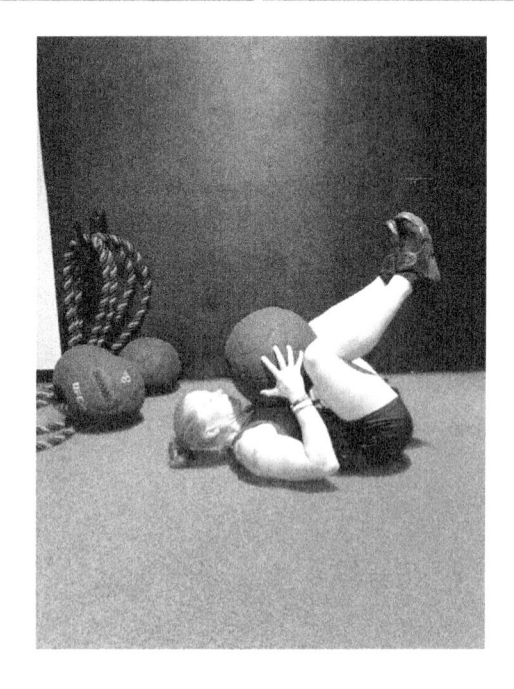

Squat rockers: Squat rockers test your coordination. This is a lower body exercise that also engages the core and stabilizer muscles. These are tough and may require some practice to stabilize yourself.

Primary muscles: Glutes, quads

Secondary muscles: Core

Steps:

1. Start with feet slightly wider than shoulder-width apart, holding the medicine ball in both hands at chest level.
2. Hinge at the hips and bend at the knees, squatting low enough to touch your elbows to your knees.
3. Let your momentum bring you all the way to the floor, bum first.
4. Keeping your knees bent, rock back on your shoulders and then rock forward again with enough momentum to bring you back onto your feet.
5. Pressing through the legs, lift yourself out of the deep squat position into a standing position (note: use your momentum from the rocker and the weight of the medicine ball to propel yourself onto your feet and up again).
6. Repeat.

DEAD BUGS

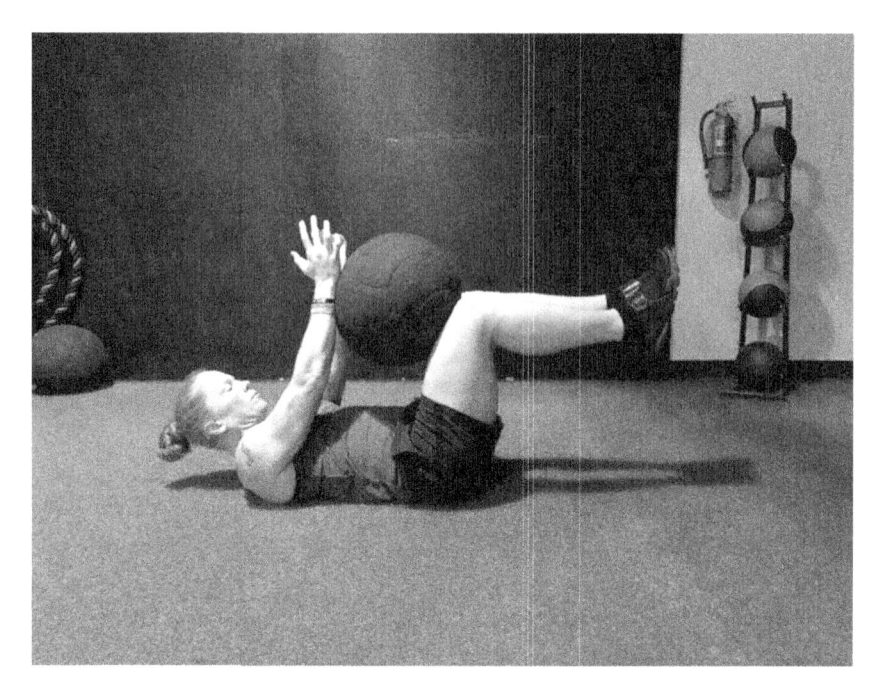

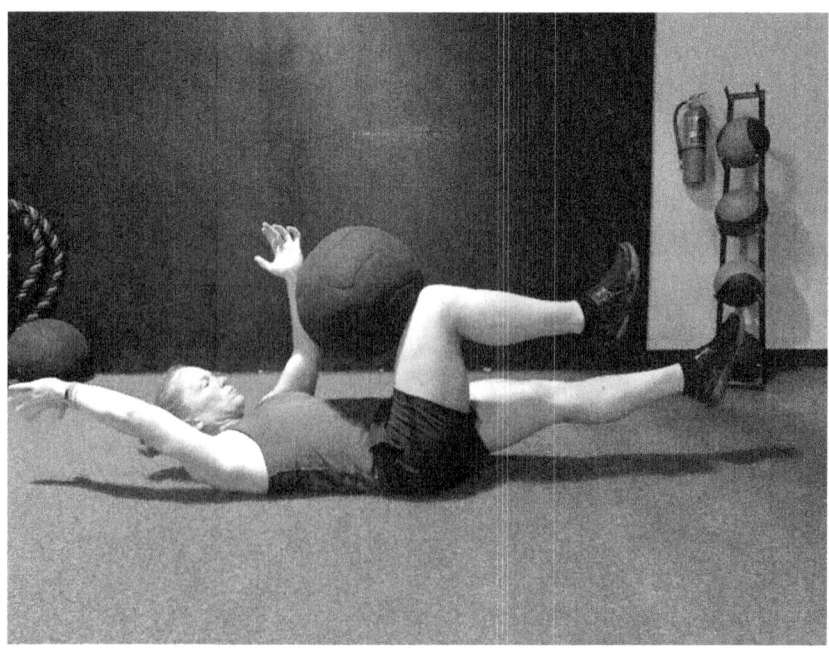

Deadbugs: By itself, the deadbug is a great core exercise. When you use a medicine ball, you force your core to be engaged at all times through the movement, and you recruit the upper and lower body to keep the medicine ball in place.

Primary muscles: Core

Secondary muscles: Lats, hamstrings

Chapter 8
8-Week Workout Program

In this workout program, you are going to see a warm-up and then the exercises. It is very important to do the warm-ups. You do not want to start your exercises with cold muscles. This can lead to injury. When you warm-up your muscles, you get blood flowing to the capillaries, tendons and the muscles, and this helps you stay free from injury.

Since many of the warm-ups repeat, we will go over the warm-ups before laying out the medicine ball exercise plan.

You can refer back here for abbreviations.

At the end of the workout plan, there's a chart where you can record your progress. You may want to make copies of this to have them for future reference

Exercise Descriptions

Wideouts—This is a lower body, plyometric exercise. Plyometrics, or jump training, are exercises that increase athletic power and explosion.

Primary muscles: Quads, glutes

Secondary muscles: Hamstrings, calves

Steps:

1. Start in a natural standing position.
2. Jump out to a wide (sumo) stance, and in a fluid motion, perform a squat.
3. As you raise yourself out of the squat position, jump back into the standing position.
4. Repeat.

Keys: This is a fluid exercise. It should be performed continuously, without stopping and starting.

Single Leg Bridge—The single leg bridge is a great bodyweight exercise for the glutes and hamstrings. You can add weight for extra resistance.

Primary muscles: Glutes, hamstrings

Secondary muscles: Abs, lower back (core)

Steps:

1. Start in a supine position (on your back) with your knees bent.
2. Straighten the right leg, keeping the left bent, so that your thighs run parallel.
3. Push through the left leg, engaging your core and squeezing the glutes, to raise your hips. Your shoulders, arms, and left leg should be the only things touching the floor.
4. Lower your body back to the floor and repeat.
5. Repeat for the right leg.

Keys: Engage the core and squeeze the glutes so that you don't sway at the hips. Your straightened leg and body should be a straight line.

Curtsy Lunge—The curtsy lunge is a lunge variation that hits the glutes hard, specifically the abductors. Do this exercise with or without added resistance (barbell, dumbbells, etc.).

Primary muscles: Glutes (abductor), quads

Secondary muscles: Calves, hamstrings

Steps:

1. Start in a natural standing position.

2. Sweep the right leg back and diagonally to the left, and plant the foot on the ground.

3. Squat down into the lunge position.

4. Push down through the left outstretched leg to raise up, and bring the right leg back to standing position.

5. Repeat with the left leg.

Keys: This lunge variation looks the way it sounds—like a curtsy. Keep the back straight and core engaged. Be sure that the knee doesn't track beyond the toe on the lunge motion.

Single Leg RDL—This exercise can be used as a stretch and a resistance movement. It primarily works the hamstrings, but is also a great exercise for balance and stability. Add resistance in the form of dumbbells, barbells, or plates to work on strength.

Primary muscles: Hamstrings, glutes

Secondary muscles: Calves, lower back muscles

Steps:

1. Start in a natural standing position.

2. With the knees slightly bent, lift the left leg off the ground and bend over, reaching back with the left leg.

3. Keep the back straight as you reach back with the leg and bend until your body forms a T shape (torso parallel with floor).

4. Return to standing position and repeat with the right leg.

Keys: Keep the back straight. Flex the glute to extend the hip. Keep the hips square; don't twist. Keep your weight close to the shin, and use controlled movements.

Inverted Row—This is a great exercise for the muscles of the back. You can make the inverted row as challenging as you'd like, so it is perfect for any fitness level. You'll need some equipment for this one.

Primary muscles: Lats, traps

Secondary muscles: Biceps, core

Steps:

1. Using a barbell set up low on a squat rack (about hip height), a TRX, or anything stable that will support your bodyweight, position yourself in a supine position under the barbell.
2. Keeping your body in a rigid, straight line (ankles, knees, hips, and shoulders in line), reach up and grab the barbell.
3. Pull yourself up high enough so that your chest touches the barbell (body still straight).
4. Lower and repeat.

Keys: Keep the core engaged and the body in a straight line—ankles, knees, hips, and shoulders in line. You can modify the exercise, to make it easier, by bending the knees.

Bird Dog—An exercise that is great for functional movement, the bird dog recruits a number of muscles. It can be done with or without resistance, and helps improve movement and core strength.

Primary muscles: Glutes, lats, shoulders

Secondary muscles: Hamstrings, core

Steps:

1. Start on your hands and knees.
2. Raise and reach with the right arm, while simultaneously raising and reaching with the left leg.
3. Extend both arm and leg, squeezing the glutes, lats, and shoulders.
4. Return to all-fours-position.
5. Repeat for left arm and right leg.

Keys: Back should remain straight—no sway and no arch. Extend through the spine and squeeze the muscles. Keep the core engaged.

Plank Ups—This is an exercise that hits the upper body as well as the core. It's a cross between a plank and a pushup.

Primary muscles: Pecs, core

Secondary muscles: Shoulders, triceps

Steps:

1. Start in a plank position (prone, resting on elbows and feet).
2. Push through your left elbow and shift your weight to the hand.
3. Push through the right elbow and shift your weight to the hand (you should now be in a pushup position).
4. Lower back to the left elbow, and then the right.
5. Repeat.

Keys: Keep the back straight and core engaged. Switch the hand you lead with (go up on the left hand then right, and then on the next rep, go right then left).

Toe Touches—Toe touches are simple to perform, but they force the abdominals to do some hard work. You'll also have to work to keep your legs in the air.

Primary muscles: Abdominals

Secondary muscles: Legs

Steps:

1. Lie flat on your back on the floor.
2. Keeping your legs straight, raise them into the air.
3. Contract the abdominals to raise your torso and touch your toes.
4. Lower your torso and repeat.

Keys: Keep the legs straight in the air. Keep the core engaged.

Alternating V-ups—This is a core exercise that recruits the legs. Core exercises that require lifting the legs are very effective at engaging the abdominal muscles.

Primary muscles: Core (abdominals and obliques)

Secondary muscles: Legs

Steps:

1. Lie flat on your back on the floor.
2. Raise the right leg straight into the air while simultaneously engaging the core to lift the torso.
3. With your left hand, touch the extended right foot.
4. Return to lying position.
5. Repeat with left leg and right arm.

Keys: Keep the legs straight when you raise them. Touch as high up on the leg as possible (toe is ideal).

Bicycle—The bicycle is another core exercise that recruits the legs. It is an active exercise requiring a lot of movement.

Primary muscles: Core (abdominals and obliques)

Secondary muscles: Legs

Steps:

1. Lie on your back with feet slightly elevated and hands behind head.
2. Bend the right knee and bring it to your chest.
3. Engage your core and touch your left elbow to the right knee.
4. Extend the right leg and bend the left, bringing the knee to the chest.
5. Touch the right elbow to the left knee.
6. Repeat quickly.

Keys: Make quick movements (like riding a bicycle). Try to touch the elbow to knee every time, twisting the torso.

Hip Series—This is a series of exercises that will engage and open the hips. Use this hip series to warm up the hip joint and all of the surrounding muscles. The series consists of hip circles (forward and back), fire hydrant, and donkey kick.

Primary muscles: Muscles around the hips (adductors, abductors, hip flexors, etc.)

Secondary muscles: Core

Steps:

1. Start on all fours and perform repetitions for the following: forward hip circles, backward hip circles, fire hydrant, and donkey kick.
2. Forward hip circles: Lift one leg and rotate at the hip joint, moving the knee forward each time. Repeat for the other leg.
3. Backward hip circles: Lift one leg and rotate at the hip joint, moving the knee backward each time. Repeat for the other leg.
4. Fire hydrant: Keeping the knee bent, lift one leg out to the side, trying to get the knee even with your back (like a dog lifting his leg on a fire hydrant). Repeat for the other leg.
5. Donkey kick: Fully extend one leg backward, squeezing the glutes (like a donkey's kick). Repeat for the other leg.

Keys: Keep the back straight and core engaged throughout each movement. Try to keep the hips square, and don't lift them.

Lunge into Hamstring Stretch—This is essentially two stretches in one: the lunge and a hamstring stretch.

Primary muscles: Glutes, quads, hamstrings

Secondary muscles: Calves

Steps:

1. Start in a full, extended lunge, right leg forward.
2. Raise your hands straight overhead, and push the hips forward, leaning into the lunge stretch. Hold for 10-15 seconds.
3. Lean back onto the left leg, straightening the right leg (extended forward).
4. Keeping the back straight, lean the torso over the extended right leg and reach for the right toe. Hold for 10-15 seconds.
5. Repeat for the left leg.

Keys: Push the hips forward and extend the arms up and back on the lunge stretch. Keep the back straight (not rounded) on the hamstring stretch.

Sumo with Torso Twist—Another combination stretch, the sumo with torso twist opens the hips while incorporating a spinal twist.

Primary muscles: Muscles around the hips, thoracic spine muscles

Secondary muscles: Chest, core

Steps:

1. Start in a wide and low sumo stance.

2. Keeping your feet on the floor (especially the heels) and the back straight, place your palms on the floor between your legs.

3. Reach up, above your head with your right arm, twisting the spine, and look up at the extended hand.

4. Return the palm to the ground and repeat for the left arm.

Keys: Keep your back straight and your heels on the ground. Sink your butt down into the squat to open the hips. Hold on the reach.

Child's Pose—The child's pose is a yoga pose that is wonderful for opening the hips. Yoga practitioners call it a restorative pose, as it helps alleviate lower back pain and overall stiffness.

Primary muscles: Hips (inner thigh), low back

Secondary muscles: Shoulders, quads

Steps:

1. Start with your legs tucked under you, about shoulder-width apart, sitting upright on your heels.

2. Bend forward at the hips, reaching with the arms and touching the forehead to the floor.

3. Extend the spine as you reach, holding the pose and breathing into the stretch.

4. Hold for at least five breaths. Repeat if needed.

Keys: Press the torso down toward the floor, into the hips. As you reach forward, try to elongate the spine.

Lunge with Torso Twist—Yet another combination stretch, the lunge with a torso twist will stretch the quads, hips and muscles along the spine.

Primary muscles: Hip muscles, quads, thoracic spine muscles

Secondary muscles: Core, glutes

Steps:

1. Start in a natural standing position.
2. Step out with the right leg, bending at the knee, into a lunge.
3. Keeping your back straight, twist your torso to the right so that your left elbow crosses your right leg.
4. Twist back to a forward-facing position and return to standing.
5. Repeat with the left leg.

Keys: Keep the back straight and core engaged. Step out far enough so that you're feeling a stretch in quad of the leg that stays back.

Thread the Needle with Reach—This is another yoga pose, with a reach added to give you another benefit. It is a great upper body stretch, and the reach adds a little spinal twist.

Primary muscles: Shoulders, chest, back

Secondary muscles: Thoracic spine muscles

Steps:

1. Start on all fours.
2. Extend the right arm straight out in the air.
3. Slide the left arm under the right and reach to the right until the left shoulder and the left side of the head are on the floor (thread the needle). Hold for 10-15 seconds.
4. Put your right elbow on the ground and bring the left arm from under the right.
5. With the left arm, reach toward the ceiling, opening the chest, and look up to your hand. Hold for 10-15 seconds.
6. Return to all fours and repeat for the other side.

Keys: Keep the palm of the extended arm on the floor. The hips shouldn't move from their original position. The gaze always follows the arm that reaches through the "needle hole."

Swimmer Arm Swings—This stretch is also known as "hug the world/hug yourself," and it is the stretch you see swimmers doing at the start of their races.

Primary muscles: Chest, shoulders, back

Secondary muscles: Spinal muscles, biceps, triceps

Steps:

1. Start in a natural standing position.
2. Quickly open your arms wide, as if you were about to hug someone (hug the world), and let your momentum stretch the chest and shoulders.
3. Close your arms quickly around yourself (hug yourself), allowing your momentum to stretch your back.
4. Repeat quickly.

Keys: This stretch should be performed with quick movements, allowing the momentum of your swinging limbs to produce the stretch.

Calf Raises—This is a simple exercise that hits an often-neglected part of the body: the calves. All you need to perform calf raises is a small step.

Primary muscles: Calves

Secondary muscles: Glutes, hamstrings

Steps:

1. Start standing on a step with toes on the step, heels hanging off.
2. Keeping the legs straight, lower the heels over the side of the step, keeping balanced on the toes.
3. Press through the toes and lift the heels up again.
4. Repeat.

Keys: Keep the legs straight and the core tight. Lower the heels enough so that you feel a slight stretch in the calf muscles.

Single Leg Squat to Box—A single leg squat to box may look simple, but it requires proper movement and a bit of strength. It's one of those exercises that is certainly harder than it looks.

Primary muscles: Glutes, quads

Secondary muscles: Hamstrings, core

Steps:

1. Stand a few inches in front of a box that's around knee-height, facing away from the box.
2. Lift the left leg slightly; keeping the back straight, squat on the right leg, until you're sitting on the box.

3. Press through the right leg, squeezing the glutes and lift yourself up from the box.

4. Repeat with the left leg.

Keys: Keep the back straight and the core engaged throughout the movement. Your weight should be on your heels when squatting.

Spiderman Plank—The Spiderman plank is a great core exercise. It is an active version of a plank, in which you bring your knees to your elbows.

Primary muscles: Core

Secondary muscles: Shoulders, legs

Steps:

1. Start on the floor, prone, on your toes and elbows (in a plank).

2. Lift the right foot off the floor, and keeping a straight back, bring the knee to the right elbow.

3. Return the foot to the floor.

4. Repeat for the left leg, all the while keeping the core engaged.

Keys: Don't let the back sway or round. Keep it straight at all times. Keep the core engaged.

Hurdle Walk—This exercise can be used to warm up the hips. Or, you can make it more active, with a hop, for some plyometric training.

Primary muscles: Muscles around hips, glutes

Secondary muscles: Core, legs

Steps:

1. Start in a natural standing position.
2. As if stepping over a hurdle, lift your right leg up and slightly to the side.
3. Step over the imaginary hurdle.
4. Lift the left leg and step over as well.
5. Repeat, leading with the left leg.

Keys: Keep the torso upright when stepping. Engage the core. The goal is to mobilize the hips, so it's not just a step. Use hip rotation.

Box Runner—The box runner is an agility drill used in speed training. It is simple enough for any fitness level and can be used in short bursts, in interval training.

Primary muscles: Glutes, hamstrings

Secondary muscles: Quads, calf

Steps:

1. Start facing a box 6-12 inches tall.
2. Quickly step up with the right foot and step down quickly.
3. As you're stepping down with the right, step up with the left, in a running motion.
4. Continue to run up on the box for a set amount of time/reps.

Keys: Use a natural running arm swing with this movement. Keep the core engaged and the torso upright, as when running.

Jump Squat—Another plyometric exercise, the jump squat utilizes the explosive power in your legs. This is another good exercise for interval training.

Primary muscles: Glutes, quads

Secondary muscles: Hamstrings, calf

Steps:

1. Start standing, with feet about shoulder-width apart.
2. Hinge with the hips and sit back into a squat.
3. Jump out of the squat explosively.
4. Land and repeat.

Keys: Engage the core throughout the movement. Keep the back straight and keep the weight in the heels during the squat.

Skaters—Skaters are performed just as they sound. This is another plyometric exercise and another good exercise for interval training.

Primary muscles: Glutes, quads

Secondary muscles: Hamstrings, calves

Steps:

1. Start standing on the right leg.
2. Bend slightly at the knee, and jump laterally to the left.
3. Land on the left foot.
4. Repeat, jumping off the left foot and landing on the right.

Keys: Stick the landing each time, working on balance and core strength. Engage the core. Jump explosively.

Arm Rotations—This is a great warm-up exercise. Arm rotations will help to loosen up the shoulders and surrounding muscles, like the pectorals.

Primary muscles: Shoulders, pecs

Secondary muscles: Back muscles, neck

Steps:

1. Start standing, with arms outstretched at shoulder height.
2. Rotate in small circles forward at the shoulder for a set time/reps.

3. Rotate in small circles backward.

4. Repeat with larger circles.

Keys: Keep the arms straight. Engage the core. The movement should be controlled.

Bear Crawl—The bear crawl is a total body exercise. Use your lower body to propel and your upper body to stabilize and guide.

Primary muscles: Glutes, hamstrings, shoulders

Secondary muscles: Pectorals, quads, core

Steps:

1. Start on all fours with the knees bent and off the ground and the back level.

2. Engage the core and crawl forward.

3. Keep the back straight and hips down as your crawl for a set time/length.

Keys: Keep the hips square, and don't open them. Engage the core and squeeze the glutes to crawl forward. Try to keep the shins parallel to the floor.

Inchworm Pushups—An upper body exercise that doubles as a lower body stretch, inchworm pushups are great for shoulder and chest strength.

Primary muscles: Shoulders, pecs

Secondary muscles: Hamstrings, calves

Steps:

1. Start by bending at the hips, keeping the legs straight (a slight knee bend is okay).
2. Place your hands on the ground; while keeping your back straight, walk yourself out to an extended position (pushup position).
3. Bending at the elbows, lower yourself to the ground and perform a pushup.
4. Keeping the knees as straight as possible, walk the feet back to the hands.
5. Repeat.

Keys: Keep the back and knees straight. Don't sway or arch during the pushup. Engage the core.

Alternating Superman—This is a variation of the Superman, in which you only raise one arm and one leg. The alternating Superman is a great low back and core exercise.

Primary muscles: Low back, core

Secondary muscles: Glutes, shoulders

Steps:

1. Start lying face down on the floor (prone), with arms and legs extended lengthwise.
2. Simultaneously lift the right and left leg off the ground, squeezing the glutes and engaging the core.
3. Lower the arm and leg.
4. Repeat with left arm and right leg.

Keys: Squeeze the glutes to lift the legs. Engage the shoulders and core to lift the arms.

Abbreviations

OH = overhead

BW = bodyweight

SL = single leg

RD = Romanian deadlift

"=seconds

Phase 1

Repeat These Workouts for Weeks 1-3

DAY 1 – Total Body (Lower Focus)

WARM-UP:

Hip Series: 5 repetitions

Lunge into Hamstring Stretch: 5 repetitions

Sumo with Torso Twist: 10 repetitions

Repeat 1 time

EXERCISE:

Medicine Ball Lunge: 3 sets x 10 repetitions each

Medicine Ball Slams: 3 sets x 12 repetitions each

Wide Outs: 3 sets x 12 repetitions each

Medicine Ball Overhead Squat: 3 sets x 12 repetitions each

Bodyweight Single Leg Bridge: 3 sets x 10 repetitions each

Bodyweight Curtsey Lunge: 3 sets x 10 repetitions each

Bodyweight Single Leg Romanian Deadlift: 3 sets x 10 repetitions each

Medicine Ball Superman: 3 sets x 12 repetitions each

Medicine Ball Woodchopper: 3 sets x 10 repetitions each

NOTES:

Hip Series = hip circle forward, hip circle back, fire hydrant, and donkey kick

Wide Outs = start standing. Hop into a wide squat position.

Hop back to standing.

DAY 2 – Total Body (Upper Body Focus)

WARM-UP

Child Pose: 30" each round

Lunge with Torso Twist: 5 repetitions each round

Thread the Needle with Reach: 10 repetitions each round

Repeat

EXERCISE:

Medicine Ball Pushups: 3 sets x 12 repetitions each

Inverted rows: 3 sets x 12 repetitions each

Medicine Ball Shoulder Press: 3 sets x 12 repetitions each

Medicine Ball Chest Press: 3 sets x 12 repetitions each

Medicine Ball V-ups: 3 sets x 12 repetitions each

Bird Dog: 3 sets x 10 repetitions each

Medicine Ball Thruster: 3 sets x 12 repetitions each

Plank Ups: 3 sets x 20 repetitions each

Medicine Ball Overhead Pass: 3 sets x 12 repetitions each

NOTE:

Plank Ups = start in a plank with elbows on the ground. Put one hand on the ground, press up to bring the other hand on the ground. From plank with hands on ground, lower back to elbows one arm at a time. Repeat.

DAY 3 – Total Body (Core Focus)

WARM-UP

Hip Series: 3 repetitions each round

Swimmer Arm Swings: 10 repetitions each round

Sumo with Torso Twist: 10 repetitions each round

Repeat 2 times

EXERCISE

Medicine Ball Lunge with Twist: 3 sets x 10 repetitions each

Medicine Ball Side Toss: 3 sets x 10 repetitions each

Toe Touches: 3 sets x 15 repetitions each

Medicine Ball Overhead Lat Bends: 3 sets x 10 repetitions each

Medicine Ball Sit-ups: 3 sets x 15 repetitions each

Alternative V-ups: 3 sets x 10 repetitions each

Medicine Ball Halo Slams: 3 sets x 12 repetitions each

Medicine Ball Russian Twist: 3 sets x 20 repetitions each

Bicycle: 3 sets x 20 repetitions each

NOTE:

Swimmer Arm Swings = swing arm wide, stretching the chest (hug the world). Swim arms around your body, stretching the back (hug yourself).

Sumo with Torso Twist = in a sumo squat, place hands on the ground. Reach with one hand to the sky. Repeat.

DAY 4 – Stair Workout (Optional)

WARM-UP

Hip Series: 5 repetitions each

Lunge with Torso Twist: 5 repetitions each

Calf Raises: 15 repetitions each

Repeat 2 times

EXERCISE

Divided into 4 blocks. Take a 45-second rest after each block.

    I.   Walking: 3 min
           Jogging: 2 min
           Rest 45 seconds

    II.   Single Leg Hops: 1 min each
           Hops: 1 min
           Jogging: 2 min
           Rest 45 seconds

    III.   Hop and Squat: 2 min
           Skip a step: 1 min
           Jogging: 2 min
           Rest 45 seconds

    IV.   2 min

Phase II

Repeat These Workouts for Weeks 5-7

DAY 1 – Low Body and Core Focus

WARM-UP

(Done as a circuit; 2 rounds)

Hip Series: 5 repetitions each

Lunge with Torso Twist: 5 repetitions each

Single Leg Squat to Box: 5 repetitions each

EXERCISE

Medicine Ball Lunge with Twist: 3 sets x 10 repetitions

Medicine Ball Thruster: 3 sets x 12 repetitions

Alternative V-Ups: 3 sets x 10 repetitions

Medicine Ball Lunge Slam: 3 sets x 12 repetitions

Medicine Ball Superman: 3 sets x 12 repetitions

Medicine Ball Deadbugs: 3 sets x 20 repetitions

Medicine Ball Overhead Squat: 3 sets x 12 repetitions

Medicine Ball V-ups: 3 sets x 12 repetitions

Medicine Ball Woodchopper: 3 sets x 10 repetitions

DAY 2 – Upper Body and Core Focus

WARM-UP

(Done as a circuit; 2 rounds)

Swimmer Arm Swings: 10 repetitions each

Sumo with Torso Twist: 10 repetitions each

Thread the Needle: 10 repetitions each

EXERCISE

Medicine Ball SA Chest Pass: 3 sets x 10 repetitions

Medicine Ball Halo Slams: 3 sets x 12 repetitions

Plank Ups: 3 sets x 20 repetitions

Medicine Ball Staggered PU: 3 sets x 12 repetitions

Medicine Ball Side Toss: 3 sets x 10 repetitions

Medicine Ball Russian Twist: 3 sets x 20 repetitions

Medicine Ball Overhead Pass: 3 sets x 12 repetitions

Spiderman Plank: 3 sets x 20 repetitions

Medicine Ball Overhead Lat Bends: 3 sets x 10 repetitions

NOTES

Spiderman Plank = plank position with elbows on ground, bring one knee to the elbow. Return and repeat with the other leg.

DAY 3 – Low Body and Movement Focus

WARM-UP

(Done as a circuit; 2 rounds)

Hip Series: 5 repetitions each round

Hurdle Walk: 10 repetitions each round

Single Leg Romanian Deadlift: 5 repetitions each round

EXERCISE

Medicine Ball Overhead Walk Lunge: 3 sets x 10 repetitions each

Wide Outs: 3 sets x 12 repetitions each

Mountain Climb Ballers: 3 sets x 20 repetitions each

Medicine Ball Squat Rockers: 3 sets x 12 repetitions each

Box Runner: 3 sets x 20 repetitions each

Bodyweight Jumper Squat: 3 sets x 12 repetitions each

Medicine Ball Burpee Wall Ball: 3 sets x 10 repetitions each

Skaters: 3 sets x 12 repetitions each

Bodyweight Curtsey Lunge: 3 sets x 10 repetitions each

NOTES

Hurdle Walk = picture walking over a hurdle. Bring knee up and over the imaginary hurdle.

DAY 4 – Upper Body and Movement Focus
WARM-UP

(Done as a circuit; 2 rounds)

Arm Rotations: 10 repetitions each round

Thread the Needle: 10 repetitions each round

Childs Pose: 30" each round

EXERCISE

Medicine Ball In and Out PU: 3 sets x 12 repetitions each

Medicine Ball Burpee Slam: 3 sets x 10 repetitions each

Bear Crawl (forward and back): 3 sets x 10 repetitions each

Medicine Ball Chest Pass to PU: 3 sets x 10 repetitions each

Inverted Row: 3 sets x 12 repetitions each

Medicine-Ball Alternating PU: 3 sets x 12 repetitions each

Medicine Ball SS Chest Pass: 3 sets x 12 repetitions each

Inchworm Pushup: 3 sets x 8 repetitions each

Alt. Superman: 3 sets x 10 repetitions each

NOTES

Alt. Superman = alternating superman. Opposite arm and leg.

Deload Week

Workout for Week 4 and Week 8

DAY 1 – Total Body (Lower Focus)

WARM-UP

(Done as a circuit; 2 rounds)

Hip Series: 5 repetitions each

Lunge into Hamstring Stretch: 5 repetitions each

Sumo with Torso Twist: 10 repetitions each

EXERCISE

Medicine Ball Overhead Walk Lunge: 3 sets x 10 repetitions each

Medicine Ball Burpee Slam: 3 sets x 12 repetitions each

Medicine Ball Woodchopper: 3 sets x 10 repetitions each

Medicine Ball Overhead Squat: 3 sets x 12 repetitions each

Medicine Ball Superman: 3 sets x 12 repetitions each

Medicine Ball Squat Rockers: 3 sets x 12 repetitions each

DAY 2 – Total Body (Upper Focus)

WARM-UP

(Done as a circuit; 2 rounds)

Childs Pose: 30" each round

Lunge with Torso Twist: 5 repetitions each

Thread the Needle with Reach: 10 repetitions each

EXERCISE

Medicine Ball Staggered PU: 3 sets x 12 repetitions

Medicine Ball Thruster: 3 sets x 12 repetitions

Medicine Ball Side Toss: 3 sets x 10 repetitions

Medicine Ball Chest Pass PU: 3 sets x 8 repetitions

Medicine Ball Wall Ball: 3 sets x 12 repetitions

Medicine Ball In and Out PU: 3 sets x 12 repetitions

DAY 3 – Total Body (Core Focus)

WARM-UP

Hip Series: 5 repetitions each round

Swimmer Arm Swings: 10 repetitions each round

Sumo with Torso Twist: 10 repetitions each round

EXERCISE

Medicine Ball Lunge with Twist: 3 sets x 10 repetitions each

Medicine Ball Dead Bugs: 3 sets x 20 repetitions each

Medicine Ball Halo Slam: 3 sets x 12 repetitions each

Medicine Ball Overhead Lat Bends: 3 sets x 10 repetitions each

Medicine Ball Sit-ups: 3 sets x 15 repetitions each

Medicine Ball V-ups: 3 sets x 12 repetitions each

NOTE (For All Days)

Deload week is a light week after a couple cycles of intense training. It's not an off week but a rest week. It's designed to keep you active but give you a break.

Medicine Ball Workout

DAY 1 – Total Body (Lower Focus)
Warm-up (done as a circuit) 2 rounds

Hip Series	x5ea
Lunge into hamstring stretch	x5ea
Sumo w/torso twist	x10

EXERCISE	REPS	WK 1	WK 2	WK 3
MB OH walk lunge	10ea			
	10ea			
	10ea			
MB burpee slam	12			
	12			
	12			
MB woodchopper	10ea			
	10ea			
	10ea			
MB OH squat	12			
	12			
	12			
MB superman	12			
	12			
	12			
MB squat rockers	12			
	12			
	12			

NOTES (on all)
Deload week is a light week after a couple of cycles of intense training. It's not an off week, but a rest week. It's designed to keep you active but give you a break.

DAY 2 – Total Body (Upper Focus)
Warm-up (done as a circuit) 2 rounds

Childs pose	x30"
Lunge w/torso twist	x5ea
Thread the needle w/reach	x10ea

EXERCISE	REPS	WK 1	WK 2	WK 3
MB staggered PU	12			
	12			
	12			
MB Thruster	12			
	12			
	12			
MB side toss	10ea			
	10ea			
	10ea			
MB chest pass PU	8			
	8			
	8			
MB Wall Ball	12			
	12			
	12			
MB in & out PU	12			
	12			
	12			

DAY 3 – Total Body (Core Focus)
Warm-up (done as a circuit) 2 rounds

Hip Series	x5ea
Swimer arm swings	x10
Sumo w/torso twist	x10

EXERCISE	REPS	WK 1	WK 2	WK 3
MB Lunge w/twist	10ea			
	10ea			
	10ea			
MB Dead bugs	20			
	20			
	20			
MB halo slam	12			
	12			
	12			
MB OH lat bends	10ea			
	10ea			
	10ea			
MB situps	15			
	15			
	15			
MB v-ups	12			
	12			
	12			

8-Week Workout Program

DAY 1 – Lower Body & core focus
Warm-up (done as a circuit) 2 rounds

Hip Series	x5ea
Lunge w/torso twist	x5ea
S. squat to box	x5ea

EXERCISE	REPS	WK 1	WK 2	WK 3
MB lunge w/twist	10ea			
	10ea			
	10ea			
MB thruster	12			
	12			
	12			
Alternating v-ups	10ea			
	10ea			
	10ea			
MB lunge slam	12			
	12			
	12			
MB Superman	12			
	12			
	12			
MB Deadbugs	20			
	20			
	20			
MB OH squat	12			
	12			
	12			
MB v-ups	12			
	12			
	12			
MB Woodchopper	10ea			
	10ea			
	10ea			

DAY 2 – Upper Body & core focus
Warm-up (done as a circuit) 2 rounds

Swimmer arm swings	x10
Sumo w/torso twist	x10
Thread the needle	x10ea

EXERCISE	REPS	WK 1	WK 2	WK 3
MB SA chest pass	10ea			
	10ea			
	10ea			
MB Halo slams	12			
	12			
	12			
Plank ups	20			
	20			
	20			
MB staggered PU	12			
	12			
	12			
MB side toss	10ea			
	10ea			
	10ea			
MB Russian twist	20			
	20			
	20			
MB OH pass	12			
	12			
	12			
Spiderman plank	20			
	20			
	20			
MB OH toe bends	10ea			
	10ea			
	10ea			

NOTES:
Spiderman plank – plank position with elbows on ground, bring one knee to the elbow. Return and repeat with the other leg.

DAY 3 – Lower Body & movement focus
Warm-up (done as a circuit) 2 rounds

Hip Series	x5ea
Hurdle walk	x10ea
SL RDL	x5ea

EXERCISE	REPS	WK 1	WK 2	WK 3
MB OH walk lunge	10ea			
	10ea			
	10ea			
Wide outs	12			
	12			
	12			
Mountain climbers	20			
	20			
	20			
MB squat rockers	12			
	12			
	12			
Box Runner	20			
	20			
	20			
BW Jump squat	12			
	12			
	12			
MB Burpee wall ball	10			
	10			
	10			
Skaters	12			
	12			
	12			
BW curtsey lunge	10ea			
	10ea			
	10ea			

NOTES:
Hurdle walk – picture walking over a hurdle. Bring knee up and over the imaginary hurdle.

DAY 4 – Upper Body & movement focus
Warm-up (done as a circuit) 2 rounds

Arm rotations	x10ea
Thread the needle	x10ea
Childs pose	x30"

EXERCISE	REPS	WK 1	WK 2	WK 3
MB in & out PU	12			
	12			
	12			
MB burpee slam	10			
	10			
	10			
Bear Crawl (forward & back)	10ea			
	10ea			
	10ea			
MB Chest pass to PU	10			
	10			
	10			
Inverted Row	12			
	12			
	12			
MB alternating PU	12			
	12			
	12			
MB SS Chest pass	12			
	12			
	12			
Inchworm pushup	8			
	8			
	8			
Alt. superman	10ea			
	10ea			
	10ea			

NOTES:
Alt. superman – alternating superman. Opposite arm and leg.

Medicine Ball Workout

DAY 1 -- Total Body (Lower Focus)

Warm-up (done as a circuit) 2 rounds

Hip Series	x5ea
Lunge into hamstring stretch	x5ea
Sumo w/torso twist	x10

EXERCISE	REPS	WK 1	WK 2	WK 3
MB OH walk lunge	10ea			
	10ea			
	10ea			
MB burpee slam	12			
	12			
	12			
MB woodchopper	10ea			
	10ea			
	10ea			
MB OH squat	12			
	12			
	12			
MB superman	12			
	12			
	12			
MB squat rockers	12			
	12			
	12			

DAY 2 -- Total Body (Upper Focus)

Warm-up (done as a circuit) 2 rounds

Childs pose	x30"
Lunge w/torso twist	x5ea
Thread the needle w/reach	x10ea

EXERCISE	REPS	WK 1	WK 2	WK 3
MB staggered PU	12			
	12			
	12			
MB Thruster	12			
	12			
	12			
MB side toss	10ea			
	10ea			
	10ea			
MB chest pass PU	8			
	8			
	8			
MB Wall Ball	12			
	12			
	12			
MB in & out PU	12			
	12			
	12			

DAY 3 -- Total Body (Core Focus)

Warm-up (done as a circuit) 2 rounds

Hip Series	x5ea
Swimer arm swings	x10
Sumo w/torso twist	x10

EXERCISE	REPS	WK 1	WK 2	WK 3
MB Lunge w/twist	10ea			
	10ea			
	10ea			
MB Dead bugs	20			
	20			
	20			
MB halo slam	12			
	12			
	12			
MB OH lat bends	10ea			
	10ea			
	10ea			
MB situps	15			
	15			
	15			
MB v-ups	12			
	12			
	12			

NOTES (on all)

Deload week is a light week after a couple of cycles of intense training. It's not an off week, but a rest week. It's designed to keep you active but give you a break.

Conclusion

Now what? You finished the 8-week workout. Now you can repeat, and it will be much easier this time. Each time you go through, you will gain confidence and strength. When it becomes easy, you can move to a heavier medicine ball. You will also note that you will increase your speed in which you can do these exercises if you stay with the same weight.

Depending on your fitness goals, you can continue to work with the lighter weights and increase your speed or move to a heavier ball, which will work more on strength. Remember, when you combine strength and speed, you get power, which is an athlete's friend.

While nutrition and recovery are not in the scope of this book, be sure to fuel your body with good whole foods after your workout. It will also be important to replenish with water. Rest is important for growth. If you're feeling ill, it's best to skip a day and pick back up when you feel better.

The medicine ball is a fantastic tool, and I hope you enjoy these workouts. We always like hearing results, and we'd love to hear from you about your strength gains and how you used the medicine ball workouts in your life.

Now that you are acquainted with the medicine ball and have a myriad of all the best workouts and exercises at your fingertips, it's time to get the ball.

Excerpt from…

Fruit Infused Water Recipes:

Recipes for your water bottle infuser, pitcher or jar

Chapter 2
Some Fruits Have It and Some Don't

When it comes to infusing, some fruits naturally have what it takes to send their tasty goodness and health-filled nutrients bursting into the water upon contact. Others, like bananas for instance, do not. They will turn brown and are too thick and mushy. Some simply lose their health benefits in the mix. But don't worry, we've done the homework for you. Here's a compiled list of the best of the best fruits for infusion:

1. **Tart Cherries**

Tart cherries add yummy taste, loads of nutrients and many health benefits to your water. While cherries are one of the smallest fruits, they bring a pint-sized package of explosive resources to the table. Be sure to use the tart (sour) variety because the sweet ones are usually best when cooked.

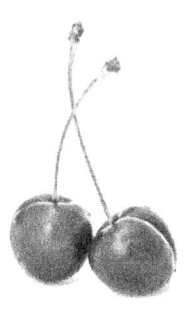

Enjoyed since around 70 B.C., cherries not only fill your glass full of flavor, they will keep your body in tip-top shape as well. They contain anthocyanins (flavonoids) that activate fat-burning molecules. Anthocyanins can boost your brain power, especially the cognitive functions, and lower your blood pressure.

These near-magical mini-fruits are bursting with benefits so potent, they are said to fight inflammation, infections and even cancer due to their high content of quercetin and ellagic, which can stop the spread and growth of tumors. In addition, they are rich in antioxidants, melatonin (for sleep), fiber and vitamins C and E. So there you have it. All that…and a cherry on top!

2. Cranberries

Another terrific tiny treat, cranberries provide a powerhouse of goodness. Cranberries are wildly popular in infusions for both taste and health benefits. Many love the slightly bitter tang of the berries, but if you are not a big fan, they can be mixed with other fruits, like cherries, so you can enjoy the nutritional value with only a hint of the flavor. On another note, cranberries have an acquired taste, so if you do blend them with another fruit, you might soon find that you really do like them after all.

Native to North America, the dark-colored berries were used by Native Americans for food and to color rugs long before the Pilgrims set foot on the land. They are rich in phenolic flavonoid phytochemicals, phenolic acids, fiber, manganese, copper and vitamins C, E and K. They are oozing with antioxidants that fight off free radicals. Free radicals cause illnesses, diseases, accelerated aging and a host of other problems. Notorious for battling away urinary tract infections, cranberries also help prevent cancer and boost the immune system.

Strawberry Mint Water

Strawberries are one of the most popular fruits for infusing. They are deliciously refreshing and are bursting with vitamins, minerals and antioxidants. Mint is a powerful pain reliever and also contains ample antioxidants, so if you want to stay healthy, this is the drink for you.

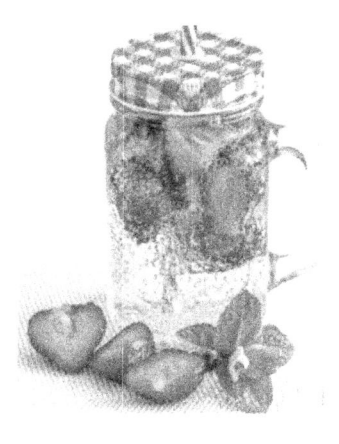

Ingredients:

- 3 cups of water
- A handful of strawberries (5-6)
- A sprig of peppermint or spearmint

Place the water in the designated compartment. Slice the strawberries and place in the fruit basket. Add the mint in with the water or in the fruit basket. Chill for several hours and enjoy.

After-Workout Infused Water Recipes

After a strenuous workout, your body needs to be replenished. Water is a must and fruits provide nutrients and minerals that are vital post-exercise as well as before. Fruits and water both help boost your energy level and help you to shed body fat while assisting in maintaining and building lean muscles. The combination also helps you to increase your metabolism. These recipes will help you to recover from all that you have put out in your workout.

Watermelon Water with Rosemary

This watermelon and rosemary-infused water drink is the ideal refreshing tonic to enjoy after a workout. It is satisfying and rewarding. Watermelon contains essential vitamins and minerals and tons of water. It adds a sweet blast to the water while rosemary brings its distinguished flavor and nutrients like calcium, iron and vitamins. Rosemary is a natural pain reliever and is awesome for the circulatory system.

Ingredients:

- 3 cups of water

- 2 slices of watermelon

- 1-2 sprigs of rosemary

Slice the watermelon into small cubes. Place the rosemary and watermelon into the fruit compartment. Add the water and drop the infuser into the water bottle. Refrigerator for at least 10 minutes before serving or longer if you wish.

Read the rest of *Fruit Infused Water Recipes* on your Kindle or in hardback at…

https://www.amazon.com/Fruit-Infused-Water-Recipes-infuser-ebook/dp/B06XV7CSF3/

Free Downloads for you

Find this book and more on Amazon.com or visit our site at 14-peaks.com for free short stories and the always free book *Click and Color*.

Printed in Great Britain
by Amazon